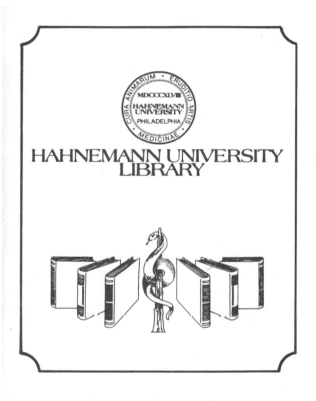

Patterns of Brief Family Therapy

The Guilford Family Therapy Series
Alan S. Gurman, *Editor*

Patterns of Brief Family Therapy

An Ecosystemic Approach

Steve de Shazer

Brief Family Therapy Center
Milwaukee, Wisconsin

Forewords by
John H. Weakland
Mental Research Institute
and
Bradford P. Keeney
Ackerman Institute for Family Therapy

The Guilford Press

New York   London

To INSOO KIM BERG,
without whom this book would not have been possible.

And to MILTON H. ERICKSON and GREGORY BATESON.
I hope they would have approved.

© 1982 The Guilford Press
A Division of Guilford Publications, Inc.
200 Park Avenue South, New York, N.Y. 10003

Printed in the United States of America
Second printing, October 1983

Library of Congress Cataloging in Publication Data

de Shazer, Steve.
   Patterns of brief family therapy.

   (The Guilford family therapy series)
   Bibliography: p.
   Includes index.
   1. Family psychotherapy.   2. Psychotherapy, Brief.
I. Title.   II. Series.
RC488.5.D4   616.89 156   81-7239
ISBN 0-89862-038-4   AACR2

Foreword
by John H. Weakland

About 25 years ago, Don D. Jackson reported to his colleagues in Gregory Bateson's research group a discovery he had made: He was not alone in sometimes seeing members of a patient's family in his psychiatric practice. Several old friends, in private get-togethers at professional meetings, had begun to reveal to him that they occasional did so too, however heretical in theory and practice as this was considered at that time. Within the next few years, family therapy, though still controversial, was clearly out of the closet. Its concepts, techniques, and application then developed quite rapidly since ideas and observations about this approach to treating problems could now be shared and discussed freely and openly.

There is a partial yet significant parallel to this in the history of brief therapy. Brief treatment has certainly been done in occasional cases by many therapists, even in psychoanalysis, all the way back to Freud himself, but it was usually done quietly and privately. Any rapid results were treated as isolated, fortuitous events—when not denigrated as "symptomatic improvement" or "flight into health"—instead of being examined and built upon. Even when brief treatment had been the subject of explicit positive consideration—a landmark being Alexander and French's 1946 work—until quite recently nearly all such considerations have cast brief therapy in a limited or a secondary role. Brief treatment has been seen as an approach of limited applicability—possibly useful in dealing with minor problems—or of limited scope—possibly useful as a bandage or stopgap in crises or in various situations where proper and thorough treatment is precluded by the circumstances. Proper and thorough treatment, of course, has meant long-term work and goals approaching rebuilding an individual or a family from the ground up.

Associated with this limited role and position assigned to brief treatment generally, has been corresponding limitations of theoretical and technical vision, even more serious in its consequences. Until recently, that is, brief treatment has largely consisted merely of "less of the same" old ideas and methods,

v

rather arbitrarily curtailed, with little concern for exploration and development of new views and approaches.

In the last few years, however, a small but growing number of therapists have begun proposing that all kinds of problems are potentially resolvable by brief treatment, and they have been exploring and describing concepts and techniques they see as relevant toward this end. Steve de Shazer's book is a significant addition to this important movement. While no written account of therapy can fully substitute for direct observation (as is true for the transmission and learning of any craft), this combination of discussion, analogies, and exemplification of the ideas and practices of de Shazer and his colleagues is more clear and specific than most books on therapy. Their work draws on and refers to much prior work, particularly that of Milton Erickson, but it also offers some novel points, such as their particular team approach and their elimination of "resistance" by redefinition as unique ways of cooperating. Moreover, even matters that may have been considered by others are presented from an angle and in a language rather special to this group.

I see all of this as positive. A view I believe Steve de Shazer and I share is that there is always change and there is no absolute truth in human affairs. Therefore, no complete, and certainly no final, account of therapy will ever be written. Meanwhile, we continue to need thoughtful and informed contributions from various perspectives. I think this book is such a contribution, one that at our present stage of knowledge and practice should be interesting and helpful to many therapists.

Foreword
by Bradford P. Keeney

Alfred North Whitehead once suggested that criticism of a book should focus on the first chapter or first page. This approach enables one to encounter the basic assumptions upon which the author's patterns of ideas are rooted. In the beginning, one's epistemological slip is always shown.

It is sometimes fashionable for family therapists to boast about their disinterest in theory or formal abstractions in favor of a more nuts-and-bolts language of therapeutic technique. Although a bit hidden, this boast is itself part and parcel of a particular epistemological position. As Gregory Bateson was fond of saying, "You cannot not have an epistemology." In fact, the idea that you do not embody an epistemology (or have any concern for such matters) may be connected to a rather bad epistemology.

Steve de Shazer's work is to be commended for beginning with an explicit statement of his epistemological position. He describes his clinical work as connected to a family of formal ideas that have been named "ecosystemic epistemology." Given this confession of orientation, he weaves stories of technique, analysis, and explanation that exemplify the way in which he and his colleagues work at the Brief Family Therapy Center.

Following an examination of de Shazer's book, some readers might ask whether parts of it are about theory, clinical practice, or research. A healthy understanding of ecosystemic epistemology would help to illuminate how that question is largely nonsense. An old idea in social science (including various psychotheologies) was that methods of clinical practice followed from formal theoretical edifices that were in turn verified by empirical (usually quantitative) research. The sequential ordering of this diachronic process was sometimes altered so that it was possible to hear that research influences clinical habit, helps to carve theory, and so on. All of these orderings embody an epistemological landscape where distinct components push and shove each other in sequential fashion (what has been called "lineal causality").

The alternative world view of "ecosystemic epistemology" organizes our experience in a more holistic fashion. Ecosystemic epistemology views research, clinical practice, and theory as inseparable and often simultaneous processes. This realization may be the most radical consequence of adopting the alternative paradigm. Pragmatically, this immediately means that one cannot exclusively reside as a clinician, researcher, or theorist. Instead, the three faces are recursively intertwined, disqualifying the knife of lineal discrimination.

Perhaps the name of such an integrated creature should be "epistemologist." Although empistemology is sometimes talked about as if it were a more philosophized package of theory, there is another way of thinking about it. The more intriguing view is to speak of epistemology as a metaphor for integrating the dissociated parts of mental process that occidentals uncritically refer to as research, clinical practice, and theory.

Along these lines, Steve de Shazer is an epistemologist. His world therefore includes strategies of intervention, elegant formalisms, and patterns of inquiry. Is it appropriate to propose that his book may be one marking of a new era in the human sciences—one that brings the epistemologist to the center of the established arenas of thought and action?

Preface

It is often difficult to know where ideas come from, and it is just as difficult to trace their development through time and space. Although an author has put ideas on paper, he or she is only responsible for that specific presentation or construction. There are two rather pertinent issues: (1) where did the ideas spring from (epistemological, theoretical, and historical roots) and (2) who *owns* the ideas.

The ideas developed in this book are historically rooted in a tradition that starts with Milton H. Erickson and flows through Gregory Bateson and the group of therapists-thinkers at the Mental Research Institute. The particular growth and development of the ideas presented in this book and the therapy described belong to a group of people who formed the core of the Brief Family Therapy Center (from here on referred to as BFTC). If new ideas can be *owned* (which is a rather peculiar, Western notion), then this group is the collective owner of the ideas. I, the author, am but a technician, a voice of the chorus. Certainly some of the ideas were built on the ideas of other therapists-thinkers; some of the ideas came out of my head and from descriptions of my work; some came from my descriptions of the work of the other core members of BFTC. All of these I helped to clarify and organize. Along with the rest of the core group I helped to create a culture in which ideas about therapy could exist, grow, develop, and be studied. But much of the historical information has been lost in the day-to-day activities of a group interested in therapy from epistemological, theoretical, and practical perspectives.

From the very beginning of BFTC, many of the ideas were developed and nurtured during informal conversations with Insoo Kim Berg and James F. Derks. Without them this book and the ideas expressed in this book would be impossible. They are both excellent therapists and teachers of therapy. I have learned a lot from watching them work with families over the years.

I owe much of this work's development to Insoo Kim Berg, my wife and colleague. Throughout she has supported my writing and thinking, sometimes at great cost to herself. I can never successfully express my appreciation.

In part to understand Insoo's heritage, my readings wandered into Asian thought. The influence of Buddhist and Taoist thought upon the epistemology and the model is central. Like Capra (13) I found the similarities between Asian thought and the new ecosystemic epistemology striking.

Working with Insoo and watching her work, I learned a lot about how to let families show us their system. She has a marvelous way of getting people to talk with each other without having to tell them to do so. Her methods have been refined and extended by the group at BFTC into what we now call our "noncritical approach."

There have been countless hours of conversation about theory and its relationship to both practice and research between Insoo and me. She probably *owns* these ideas as much as I do. I just put them on paper.

One case in 1979, where Jim Derks had been the conductor (or member of the therapy team in the room with the family), pointed out to me that we had developed a new method of relating one task to the response a family reported to the previous task. While Jim and his team worked with the family, I just watched the videotapes. I remember telling Jim that "something was different" and that he should save the tapes. After years of watching Jim's work, something struck me about the particular approach to this family's puzzle. Jim saw his step-by-step approach just as tailored to this particular family with its particular puzzle. Only later study pointed out to me the germinal nature of this new way of looking at the approach to this family: It clarified for me, and us, the methods we had developed to relate one task to another.

This is but one example, but it points out the nature of the development of ideas and the relationship of practice to model building. While I saw this approach as "different," Jim maintained it was "business as usual." I knew it was not how either of us, or Insoo, would have approached the same puzzle three years earlier. But later study of the tapes and study of tapes of other cases "proved" Jim correct. It was just business as usual: We have been working this way for more than two years.

But I too was "right." Because I saw something different, I was able to see how our model was different from what we did in the past, and a new model of therapy was born. (So, who owns these ideas?) Because we now have the apparatus available, we could watch a large number of family therapy sessions and could therefore see the patterns.

DEVELOPMENT

Our model was not born fully mature. It developed gradually over a period of time with the assistance of others beyond the core group of BFTC.

Recently it has become common practice among some family therapists and among many brief therapists to work in front of a one-way window with an observer or group of observers behind the glass. Many times this is done for training purposes (50), with the trainee in front of the glass while the trainer watches. During the session the trainer is attentive to both the family's needs and the trainee's needs. In general, the contact between trainer and trainee during the session is limited to phone calls. When the trainer wants to give advice, suggestions, or comments, he* simply calls. The trainer's job is to correct errors made right when they happened rather than waiting for a postmortem supervisory session when this error correction would be too late.

Charles Fulweiler, in a discussion with Haley and Hoffman (36), described using the mirror in a different manner; he used it while working alone. This allowed him to give a family an in-session task to perform while he went and observed. In this way he was able to minimize the direct interference of the therapist during the task. But, the setting itself was a form of interference: It was not like a candid camera technique of observing while the family was unaware. However, this technique allows the therapist to achieve a greater distance and to get a more "objective" view of the family similar to that which an observer gets while behind the mirror. It also gave the therapist some time out to think about what to do to be helpful to the family.

Some groups, like the Mental Research Institute (64, 67) and BFTC (before the development of the new model), used a group of peers behind the mirror as on-the-spot consultants. Again, most frequent contact during a session was over the phone. The group would call in suggestions when they became aware the therapist was having difficulties. Infrequently a therapist from behind the mirror would go into the therapy room for a short time to deliver this assistance. In general, the one-way window was thought of as just another part of the wall. The group and the therapist were as separate as they would have been if the wall had been solid. They would meet before and after the session to review the work and to plan future strategy and tactics.

The Consulting Break

One day while the BFTC group was seeing a family, the barrier broke down. A suggestion was called in. The therapist disagreed and so he left the room to consult with his peers. Once the disagreement was settled, a plan was jointly developed for the remainder of the session. From this beginning, a "consulting break" became routine with the group. It was seen as a vast improvement upon the telephone communication system.

---

*For the sake of simplicity and clarity, I have used throughout this book the masculine pronoun. It is, of course, understood that therapists, trainers, researchers, and clients can be male or female.

However, this change in therapist–group interaction was not immediately perceived as a *difference that made a difference* (9). In most instances, the therapist just came out to talk over his plan for the remainder of the session and to receive comments and suggestions. When the therapist was a junior member of the group the observers were likely to be more directive about the plan. But the group behind the mirror still saw themselves as "observers," there to watch other members of the group work with families. Primarily, this whole activity was seen as a chance to learn more about the practice of brief therapy.

Even though the consulting break became routine, the group continued to see the therapist and the family as "out there" and as objects of study, with the group safely separated from the therapy session by a wall. The group was acting "as if" they were part of a candid camera crew and therefore did not see themselves as interfering too much. In fact, they attempted to limit the interference as much as possible except for taking the break. The therapist, too, would behave "as if" he were working alone, except for routinely leaving the room once during the session to consult.

The Compliment

One day a client helped to change that perception. It was not long after the intervention of the consulting break when a client asked for the observers' comments. Neither the therapist nor the group was prepared for this. However, the request seemed reasonable enough. The group phoned in a short, highly complimentary statement about the family's efforts to deal with their impossible problem. The family beamed, and the therapist went ahead with his planned intervention as though nothing important had happened. The session ended on a very positive note.

Realizing it or not, something important had happened. The wall between the group and the therapy situation had broken down, in a fashion similar to that in subatomic physics:

> Nothing is more important about the quantum principle than this, that it destroys the concept of the world as "sitting out there," with the observer safely separated from it by a 20-centimeter slab of glass. Even to observe so miniscule an object as an electron, he must shatter the glass. He must reach in. He must install his chosen measuring equipment. . . . Moreover, the measurement changes the state of the electron. The universe will never be the same afterward. To describe what has happened, one has to cross out that old word "observer" and put in its place the new word "participator." In some strange sense, the universe is a participatory universe. (Wheeler, in 13, p. 127)

Shattering the glass between the therapy and the group behind the mirror soon became part of a "new therapeutic format," which eventually developed into a new model that demanded a new ecosystemic epistemology (70) and a new theory of change.

The participators behind the mirror started to work with the therapist in the room, now called the "conductor," during the consulting break to construct the major intervention as a statement from the team to the family. In general, these statements start with something phrased in a positive manner. The conductor takes this statement, called a "compliment," with him when he returns to the therapy room. The rationale for returning with a compliment is simple. Originally, these messages were designed to strengthen the team's position as the therapist became the voice of a chorus when he returned to the room. The statements are phrased in positive terms to soften the impact of the team's presence based on the assumption that the family might expect a team of experts to give the family a rough time by being critical.

For a limited time each week, the team refined this participatory approach to brief therapy. Unknown to us, a group in Milan (56) and a group in New York (5) started to behave in much the same fashion.

The participators behind the mirror started to reach into the session further as the impact of the chorus became more clear. Once BFTC became a full-time effort and this approach became more and more refined, the roles of the conductor and the participators became defined in ways that forced the team to reach further and further into the therapy session. At this point the conductor and the participators started to see themselves as a single unit, a therapy team, and then came to see the family as a subsystem of a larger suprasystem that included the therapy-team system: an ecosystemic perspective. That is, a point of view or a way of description developed that includes the system's ecological connections.

Behind the mirror, the task became to design interventions and to observe the results. In front, the task became to form a workable relationship with the family and to collect data necessary for the rest of the team behind the mirror to do their jobs. During the consulting break the results of both tasks are joined together. When the conductor returns to the therapy room, he becomes the voice of the whole team. He gives the family a carefully orchestrated set of interventions designed by the whole team.

As a result of the new format and as a result of the shift of perception about the team's role, certain concepts and theories carried over into the model from various predecessors began to fall by the wayside. Conceptual models are like any other system: If you change one element, this change will affect the other elements and the relationships between the elements in some way. This book is about those changes.

Acknowledgments

Some of the developments owe a debt to Marvin Weiner, MD. Marv was one of the cofounders of BFTC. He is a family practitioner who became interested in family therapy, and he started to treat families (in therapy) without the same psychological-sociological biases of other team members. Since he was not trained in psychopathology, he helped us to keep our focus: Family puzzles are normal attempts to handle life's many difficulties. Some just do not work.

Many hours of conversations with Elam Nunnally, Eve Lipchik, and Alex Molnar, all members of BFTC, have helped to clarify some of the ideas and to show how they differ from other models. Finally, another member of BFTC, Marilyn La Court, has been very helpful in designing the "Möbius map" (see Chapter 5) and in the theory construction derived from this work.

The therapy model described in this book was refined and explored in a culture or context involving many other people. BFTC is equipped with one-way mirrors and videotaping machines. Frequently, others beyond the core team are involved on a team behind the mirror. Among these have been various trainees and graduate students who deserve thanks for teaching BFTC how to teach this model.

Further thanks is due John Ludwig and Tom Ayers (past and present directors, respectively, of the Family Service Agency of Dundee, Illinois). My consultive relationship with their training program helped me to see the value of this model and its particular format as a teaching and training tool. Seeing the model in use by therapists other than the core group lead to an important principle: The model is independent of the therapists using it.

Various people in addition to the BFTC group have read parts of the manuscript in various forms. Some of the suggestions were useful, all were clarifying; their contributions show up in the final text. Particular thanks to Bradford Keeney, Lyman Wynne, Elliot Lipchik, Robert Peterson, and Chungja Kim.

●   ●   ●

My problem in studying therapy is that the investigator is much like this famous toad:

> The centipede was happy, quite
> Until a toad in fun
> Said, "Pray, which leg goes after which?"
> This worked his mind to such a pitch,
> He lay distracted in a ditch,
> Considering how to run.

But, I am only a centipede pretending to be a toad.

Contents

Introduction

ECOSYSTEMIC EPISTEMOLOGY

Every clinical model that is teachable and every coherent theory, be it about family therapy or physics, must have an epistemological foundation. And it is only natural that *knowing, thinking, and deciding* about family therapy should reflect the thinking of Gregory Bateson (8, 9). Ever since his early work in the field with Ruesch (4) and his subsequent work on the double-bind theory (5), Bateson's thoughts have had a large impact on the field of family therapy. As is the case in this book, Bateson's influence has been both implicit and explicit.

Since the context in which this theory and model developed is "family therapy" and because the family is generally thought of as "a system," the epistemology needs to be systemic. Wildon and others have pointed out that in "von Bertalanffy's conception, the 'environment' is in essence a kind of passive 'ground' in which the 'organism' (figure) moves" (71, p. 39). Since this was the predominant conceptualization during the growth period of many systemic models of family therapy, this description was carried over into the models and conceptualizations of family therapy.

With this conceptualization as a foundation, it is easy to commit the error of drawing a boundary between the family system and the therapist, while the behavior between the family and the therapist is fully interactive, communicative. From this perspective, however, the therapist is generally as separated from the family system as the traditional chemist in his laboratory is separated from the chemicals with which he works. Many models of *family-systems therapy*, therefore, fall into the prevailing epistemology that

> in Bateson's terms, is an epistemology of lineal causation or "force" or "power." For the general systems theorist it involves the imposition of closed-system thinking on those aspects of reality which are open systems; it denies the relationship between energy and information by splitting wholes (ecosystems) into supposedly independent "things." (71, p. 210)

This error of reifying the differences between the components of a whole into

"imaginary oppositions" (71, p. 219) can lead to attempts to apply the traditional scientific methods of research (one cause, one effect) on a system that
has circular or even more complex chains of determination.

Of course, some regularity of the relationship between cause and effect is
assumed. Without that assumption, nobody could possibly guess at the differences between cause and effect given a complex chain of causation.
"This—the fact of difference between effect and cause when both are incor-
porated into an appropriately flexible system—is the primary premise of what
we may call transforming or coding" (9, p. 110). But the traditional scientific
method of isolating one cause for one effect is inappropriately simple for a complex ecosystemic framework. Because the system, or ecosystem, "is circular,
effects of events at any point in the circuit can be carried all around to produce
changes at that point of origin" (9, p. 104).

The same boundary error clearly obtained in those models of family-
systems therapy that included an observer, or observers, behind a one-way
mirror. In general the observing group was not thought of as part of the
"therapy system" even by those who attempted to keep the therapist with the
family in the same systemic description. If a different, ecosystemic punctuation
is used that views the therapy system as an open system, then the therapist
system needs to be included in the description with the family system. Furthermore, both the therapist and the observers can be seen as part of the family-
system's environment, which (metaphorically for the field of family therapy) is
what Wheeler is talking about when he describes physicists breaking through
their glass shield with their tools, and therefore becoming participators rather
than observers: the Heisenberg Hook, which states that an observer cannot
observe without interferring with the observed. Once the description of therapy
includes the therapist's system (which includes the group behind the mirror)
and the family system, a new suprasystem needs to be considered. This way of
thinking, knowing, and deciding is called an ecosystemic epistemology (47,
70).

This epistemology has its own set of methodological boundaries around
the family and the therapists' subsystems, which are described as components
of a new suprasystem. Each subsystem, during the therapy, is part of the other
subsystem's environment or context. Since the two subsystems communicate—an attribute of an open system—their interaction becomes circular or
more complex.

> They act sequentially and simultaneously as well. In fact, people speak in
> sequence, hold talk and eyes simultaneously, and do things under a pre-
> vailing system of moods, plans, dress, insignia, decor, and setting. And
> nowadays we would not agree that participants simply cause each other to
> speak and act. We would say that the activities are also caused by the larger

contexts of each one's life, their ongoing relationship, the agenda they were following in the encounter, and larger systems of context as well . . . "communication" covers all of the things people do, say, and think together. (53, p. 131)

THE HOMEOSTASIS MUDDLE

Since the business of family therapy is change, an ecosystemic epistemology must contain the foundation for a theory of change.* The family-systems model was based on the concept of "homeostasis," a concept that included homeostatic mechanisms that were described as restoring the system to its status quo, thus keeping the patient sick (45). This interpretation of the concept of homeostasis, rather than being a systemic notion, seems mechanical; a closed loop "like Ashby's unfortunately labeled 'homeostat.' Ashby's machine is restricted to random search for stability: it has no memory and it cannot learn. It is a closed system because it is closed to information and control and open only to energy" (71, p. 375). Therefore, it is its own environment and it seeks mechanical equilibrium. As such, this concept of homeostasis, based on the homeostat, fits the more or less closed system concept of the early family-as-a-system view based on von Bertalanffy.

As the concept of homeostasis (including homeostatic mechanisms) became more generally accepted, homeostasis became equated with "nonchange," and it became one of those "ideas which handicap therapists" beyond those listed by Haley (39). In fact, a muddle developed.

Speer (59) asked: "Is homeostasis enough?" and answered: "No." A theory of stability — or, how things do not change — is not a good foundation for a theory of change, and, therefore, it is a profound irony that family therapy's conceptualizations were built on homeostasis. Speer went on to suggest adding the concept of "morphogenesis" (structure changing) to the terms of a family-systems theory. This concept had been introduced to cybernetics by Maruyama, who described morphogenesis in this way:

> Once a system is kicked in a right direction and with sufficient initial push, the deviation-amplifying mutual positive feedbacks take over the process, and the resulting development will be disproportionally large as compared with the initial kick. (48, p. 166)

The need for a concept of morphogenesis was described by Buckley:

> In dealing with the sociocultural system . . . we jump to a new system level and need yet a new term to express not only the structure-maintaining

---

*The full description of an epistemology for family therapy is beyond the scope of this book, which is primarily clinical in focus.

feature, but the structure-elaborating and changing feature of the inherently
unstable system, i.e., a concept of morphogenesis. (12, p. 15)

Hoffman (42), like Buckley, describes "the family system" as a system having
homeostatic, or morphostatic features, or levels and morphogenetic features.

However, by 1982 the question is still not settled, and Dell (17) repeats the
question: "Is homeostasis enough?" Dell critiques the current uses and misuses
of the term "homeostasis" and concludes that the term has become useless and
confusing.

What Dell and other therapists who have questioned the concept of
homeostasis have failed to realize is that "stability" and "changing" are terms of
different logical types. The class of things, events, patterns, or systems that can
be called "stable" *excludes* the class of things, patterns, or systems that can be
called "changing." Therefore, the proper answer to Speer's question comes in
two parts: (1) "Yes," homeostasis is enough on the level used to describe systemic stability; and (2) "no," homeostasis is not enough on the level used to
describe systemic change; the organizing concept on this level is "morphogenesis."

The early conceptualizers in the field were struggling to find a way to
organize their perceptions of "the family as a system." What seems to have
struck them with great force was the perceived imperviousness of troubled
families. Some ideas from cybernetics fit what they observed: families acting
"as if" they were cybernetic systems. Therefore, they borrowed the concept of
"homeostasis" to organize their observations of the *stability of these families*.
(Of course this concept readily fit with the therapeutic concept of "resistance,"
which was part of the culture in which the conceptualization of the family as a
system developed.)

Certainly the families they studied had managed to maintain their troublesome behaviors for a long time, and the concept of homeostasis gave them a
heuristic device to define and study these phenomena. Therefore, Bateson *et
al.* (6) could describe the family as an error-activated, self-correcting, homeostatic system.

What the early conceptualizers and therapists since then have failed to
realize is that "the study of the family" and "the study of family therapy" are
studies of different logical types. The former is a study of stability, while the latter is a study of changing. That is, homeostasis is a valuable concept when "the
family as a system" is the focus of study. In this situation the methodological
boundary is drawn around the system under consideration: "the family."
However, when the system under consideration is defined as "the open system
of the therapy situation," then the boundary is drawn around the therapist and
the family subsystems of the therapeutic suprasystem. Then the organizing
concept needs to be different because the focus is on *changing*: morphogenesis. Otherwise, the paradox of describing a theory of change built on a concept

of stability results: an epistemological error that necessitates conceptual gymnastics in order to explain what it is that is going on in the family therapy situation.

What seems to have happened then, is that the methodological boundary that is necessary for the study of the family as a system was carried up to the next, more complex level where this boundary became a barrier. That is, when therapy and changing were looked at with homeostasis in mind, an artificial opposition between therapist (for change) and the family (homeostatic, and therefore against change) was created because of the comparatively closed system description (the family as homeostatic system) used to describe part of, or one component of, the more open therapeutic suprasystem. Thus the "homeostasis muddle," or paradox, was created by confusing logical types.

A theory of therapeutic change necessitates a description on this more complex level (the suprasystem), and a morphogenetic or ecosystemic epistemology is appropriate for such a theory. The clearing up of the homeostasis muddle paves the way for a theory of change using the concept of morphogenesis, a theory of change that does not need conceptual gymnastics to account for stability within a theory of changing systems. Stability is not the proper focus of an epistemology suitable for family therapy, and therefore stability is not a concern for a theory of change.

CHANGE

One of the central points of Bateson's epistemology (8, 9) is the *difference that makes a difference* or an "idea" that is the *news of difference*. "In mental process, the effects of difference are to be regarded as transforms (i.e., coded versions) of the difference which preceded them" (9, p. 109). And both terms "transforms" and "difference," are words associated with the term "change." Primarily, information is a message about a difference. When Bateson says "that information is the difference which makes a difference, he is referring to that use of distinction, within any given set of variables, which makes the further and continued transformation of differences possible" (71, p. 222). Bateson describes one of the sources for an idea as developing from having two description of the same process or sequence that are differently coded or differently collected. That is, the relationship between the two descriptions is a bonus or the news of a difference.

> The first step is to recognize that *the unit of survival is the message-in-circuit in the ecosystem,* whether the ecosystem in question be methodologically defined at the biological, the sociocultural, the psychological, or at some other level. Unlike energy, information (messages) can be both created and destroyed, primarily because the very possibility of information depends

upon a code which is shared by both sender and receiver. (By "sender" and
"receiver" I mean the heuristic device which enables us to talk about the
message-in-circuit.) The code, in fact, as Bateson points out, is the relationship. Without the reciprocity of the code, the message is received as
"noise." And when the possibility of information is destroyed by the
breakdown of the sender-receiver relationship, the ecosystem perishes.
(71, p. 218)

Thus the "sender" (the therapist sub-system) of the therapeutic message needs
to share a code or a relationship with the "receiver" (the family subsystem) of
the message, otherwise the message will not get from one component of the
ecosystem to the other and the therapeutic ecosystem will perish. But that message within the "code" needs to contain information that is about a difference
that makes a difference, otherwise there will be no change. And change is, after
all, the business of therapy.

●   ●   ●

If, as Wildon maintains, all epistemological errors in science and philoso-
phy are errors of punctuation, then many of the errors of epistemology that will
be found in this text are probably errors of exactly the same type of those the
text is criticizing. This is hardly surprising given the dominance of the "old" prevailing epistemology.

CHAPTER 1

A Binocular Theory of Change*

ISOMORPHISM

Once the therapy team broke through the mirror and became participants rather than observers, it became obvious that an ecosystemic epistemology (47, 70) was necessary (see Introduction). Thus the basic elements of the therapy situation came to be seen as patterns involving the families and the therapists (or, more correctly, the therapy team) and the interaction or exchange of information between these two components of the therapeutic system. The two subsystems (family subsystem and the therapy team subsystem) can be seen to interact in such a way as to create a new pattern or patterns, and thus a suprasystem. "This view of the intertwining relational fields of the therapist and the identified patient are comparable to moire patterns where two independent patterns interact to create an emergent new pattern" (47, p.126). This fundamental change in our descriptions and observation methods implies a modification in the general structure of the therapeutic endeavor and the theory behind it, necessitating a new theory or model of change that recognizes the "impossibility" of separating the scientific observer from the observed phenomena"(13, p.266).

As the two subsets of patterns (family's subset and therapy-team's subset) become intertwined, the theory of change that guides the therapists' interventions must be based on the new pattern that is seen to develop. The theory needs to guide the description of the emergent pattern, and this pattern needs to be interactionally described. Furthermore, the description involved needs to include, first, the family's complaint pattern, then the intervention pattern, then the family's report on its response to the intervention, then the next intervention, and so on. It is necessary to include this description of the patterns that develop over the time of the therapy so that the therapy team, to some extent at least, can know the usefulness of its interventions.

---

*Thanks to Bradford Keeney for reading an earlier version of this material and for suggesting the label for the theory.

This conceptual scheme suggests that there needs to be something about the pattern of interventions and something about the family's complaint pattern and something about the interaction between these two patterns that can promote change. Two primary concepts, the *concurrent* concepts of "isomorphism and "cooperating," have developed since the therapy team became participators that can define what the "something about" seems to be and how that something about the interaction between the subsystems can effect the change process.

One of Bateson's ideas is suggestive of how this something about the emergent patterns need to be described. "If you walk around with pattern A and you encounter pattern B all you get is your pattern A and a hybrid of A and B. You never see B" (47, p. 126). Therefore, if the therapeutic intervention can be described as "pattern B" and the family's complaint pattern can be described as "pattern A," then the family will at most receive a blend of the two: A and B. It is equally true that the therapy team, walking around with pattern B and encountering the family's pattern A can never see A. The team will at most receive a blend of B and A. The difference between "blend B and A" and "blend A and B" is crucial to the binocular theory of change. If this is descriptive of what happens, then the family receiving an intervention will *never* receive the message, except as part of a hybrid. If change is going to be involved in these emergent patterns, then pattern B needs to be closely related to pattern A so that intervention can serve to reframe or redefine pattern A. The concrete facts of the situation may remain the same, but the context in which they are set may change. This is at least somewhat acceptable to the family because the intervention covers familiar territory.

The concept of isomorphism can further help to refine the definition of what the something about the patterns and the descriptions of the patterns need to include.

> The word "isomorphic" applies when two complex structures can be mapped onto each other, in such a way that to each part of one structure there is a corresponding part in the other structure, where "corresponding" means that the two parts play similar roles in their respective structures. This usage of the word "isomorphic" is derived from a more precise notion in mathematics. (43, p.49)

Hofstadter strongly suggests "that it is such perceptions of isomorphism which create *meanings* in the minds of people" (43, p.50). And, the meaning in the therapy situation can be described as "change." In general, the change process can be seen to start with an "idea," or the news of difference that is a "result" of reframing or changing the contextual meanings of a set of concrete "facts" (64). However, reframing is not an act, but a process (21) that changes the family's perception of its situation and allows for new behaviors (which demonstrates the change in perceptions) that in turn creates new subjective experiences. The concept of isomorphism suggests that if the therapy team's description and intervention pattern B is more similar to a pattern A_1 (a reframed version of the same pattern A), then the family will perceive meaning in the hybrid A and A_1, which is likely to promote change.

A metaphor about the "bonus" of depth perception that we receive from the two eyes seeing the same things *from different angles* further clarifies the something about the team's description and the intervention process. The right eye's view can be mapped onto the left eye's view *isomorphically*, and the meaning of this is the "bonus of depth perception." That is, the brain can be described as receiving two messages: (1) each eye's view of the same thing: isomorphism and (2) the "news of difference" between the views of the individual eyes: a relationship that develops depth perception. This news of difference is an important part of the epistemology behind the bincoluar theory of change and is an important part of how we know.

The concept of isomorphism can thus be applied to therapy as the ability of the team to describe the family's patterns (A) in such a way that their reframed description (A_1) can serve as a guide for designing an intervention that can be mapped onto the pattern the family has described and shown (A). The elements of the team's description need to correspond to the elements of the family's description and the patterns it has shown the team in the therapy session(s). Furthermore, the team's description (A_1) needs to be from a different angle so that the family (at least potentially) can receive the news of a difference, a perceptual shift, which promotes change in the family patterns. The resultant behavior change will create a different subjective experience. This isomorphic description enables the therapy team to design isomorphic interventions, in particular the "compliment subset" of the intervention set of "compliment and clue."

If the concept of isomorphism is used as part of the binocular theory of change without Bateson's ideas about the news of difference, there is the danger that the therapeutic error called "being sucked into the family system" may occur. This might also be described as an "accidental isomorphism" and is not useful to the family or the therapy because there is no different angle to provide the desired depth perception or bonus that leads to change.

COOPERATING

As the binocular theory of change developed, the concept of isomorphism was joined by the concurrent concept of "cooperating": *Each family (individual or couple) shows a unique way of attempting to cooperate, and the therapist's job becomes, first, to describe that particular manner to himself that the family shows and, then, to cooperate with the family's way and, thus, to promote change.* (That is, some families manner of cooperating is shown to the team to include performing tasks that will promote change. The families' manner of using tasks was previously described through the lens of resistance: Some families would do tasks, some would avoid tasks, some would modify tasks, and some would do the opposite of the tasks. Avoiding, modifying, or doing the opposite was described as "resistance." The use of tasks will be described in Chapter 4 as will the general categories of cooperating.) The definition of cooperating uses the "ing" form of the word to help remind the therapist of the process of continuing interaction between the two subsystems. The concept of cooperating seems more useful and seems to better fit an ecosystemic epistomology than did the concept of resistance, which it replaced. While the concept of isomorphism refers *mainly* to the meanings, contexts, or conceptual, emotional settings in which a situation is experienced, the concept of cooperating refers *mainly* to the concrete behaviors involved in a situation. It must be noted that these concepts are "concurrent." That is, the concepts are not used separately (i.e., *either* isomorphism *or* cooperating). Rather, the two concepts are used together (i.e., *both* isomorphism *and* cooperating). Therapeutic change involves both perceptual and behavioral changes.

Originally, the concept of resistance was part of various models of therapy and part of a different epistemology and, therefore, part of different theories of change. The concept was used to explain certain behaviors of the client who was seen as an object of study "out there." A client's behavior was explained as being the result of internal dynamics, and "resistance" was the term used to describe the client's reluctance to recover some anxiety-evoking experiences. The therapist's job was described as uncovering this repressed material, but when he touched on this area of the client's life, the client was seen to resist the therapeutic effort. This lineal concept was carried over into more interactionally described models of therapy, and the term "resistance" was also carried over, though the definition started to change.

One of the great innovators of therapeutic procedures is Milton H. Erickson. His work provided news of a difference that greatly influenced the development of family therapy and brief therapy (see Chapter 2). From his hypnotic orientation, Erickson developed a definition that expanded the term "resistance" to include some of the therapist's behavior in the situation.

> You suggest that they withhold—*and they do.* And you also suggest that they tell—*and they do.* But they withhold and they tell responsively. And as long as they are going to withhold, *you ought to encourage them* to withhold. (37, p. 97)

Since withholding can be described as a type of resistance, this concept became generalized to what might be called "Erickson's First Law": *As long as they are going to resist, you ought to encourage them to resist.* (This law was at least implicit in Erickson's work for years.)

The brief therapists at the Mental Research Institute (MRI) have based much of their work on developments of Erickson's procedures. They refined Erickson's concepts by including the therapist's reactive behaviors to the resistance to change:

> In more than one sense this form of problem resolution is similar to the philosophy and technique of judo, where the opponent's thrust is not opposed by a counterthrust of at least the same force, but rather is accepted and amplified by yielding to and going with it. This the opponent does not expect; he is playing the game of force against force, of more of the same, and by the rules of his game he anticipates a counterthrust and not a different game altogether. (64, p. 104)

Thus, the resistance is still seen as "located" in the client and is described as something the client is *doing* rather than as a *product* of client-therapist interaction. This definition of the concept of resistance is a result of splitting the ecosystem by placing the boundary between therapist and client, thus creating "imaginary oppositions" (71) between the two components of the ecosystem. The concept of cooperating instead defines these behaviors as part of the pattern of interaction between the family subsystem and the therapist, or the therapy-team subsystem.

While still using the Ericksonian definition, the group behind the mirror at BFTC devoted its efforts to figuring out ways to "encourage and utilize the resistance" to help insure that both family and therapist could have their desired outcomes. The family's resistance was seen as a natural part of its system (or subsystem) and was considered to be part of the normal "homeostatic mechanisms."

To describe more fully these homeostatic mechanisms, the author developed a model based on balance theory (20, 22). This model described the problem as being maintained by the balanced state of the relationships between and among family members despite their desire to change. The homeostatic mechanisms were seen as the balanced state of the relationships. Moreover, this model allows family interaction (the homeostatic mechanisms) to be mapped with a certain rigor and can be used to describe the current state of the family (sub)system as observed by the therapist. It also includes guidelines to help the therapist initiate change in the family from one type of organization (a certain balanced state) to another type of organization (some different balanced state); it describes situations that are imbalanced as having tendencies to move toward a balanced state. That is, the balance theoretical model includes a concept of change unlike most models built on homeostatic concepts. Once the relationships between or among the people are different, the system will tend to seek a steady state (any steady state) that is different from the preceding balanced state.

> This evolving steady state is what Bateson is describing with the term "self-healing tautology." That is, any organizationally closed system is tautologous in that each aspect of the system implies the remainder of the system. This is why one can intervene in a system at any point: If any aspect of the system is changed, the organization of the system as a whole is thereby changed. (16)

Although the relationship between the therapist and the family is discussed briefly in the balance theoretical model, the therapist is still described as viewing the clients as out there in a manner similar to Erickson or MRI. The balance theoretical model is basically a closed system model that drew a boundary between components of an ecosystem. Furthermore, the balanced states of the relationships are too easily equated with nonchange, or resistance to change, and therefore it is a poor conceptual model for family therapy.

Once the team started to become involved with families as "the therapy team," the concept of resistance was replaced by the concept of cooperating. As soon as the consulting break became the routine practice, the team noted that the term "resistance" and the phrase "utilizing and encouraging the resistance" dropped out of the vocabulary. The team, now full participators, started to send in major reframing messages (including tasks) after the consulting break. Most of these messages are phrased as coming from the team as a whole: "We are all impressed . . . " or, "We all think. . . . " The team was now involved in reaching into the therapy situation, and the family was no longer seen as out there. In this model, the therapist is *not* described as in a contest between change and nonchange because the team stopped describing the family (sub)system as resisting, or as a (sub)system stuck in concrete by homeostatic mechanisms, or as not changing because of the balanced state of relationships. Built on the concept of the ecosystem as an open system, the team's conversation started to focus on the manner in which the team expected the family to react to and cooperate with the intervention designed to promote change. The question became: What is the family showing the team about how the team might help the family accept a message that could help them move the family outside their original frame so that change can happen?

It must be kept clear that resistance is only a metaphor for describing certain regularities of phenomena, and that other metaphors can be used. Resistance is not something concrete, only a concept used as an explanatory metaphor. Resistance is only one among many ways (including cooperating) to describe what it is that the observer is observing. One can only choose a particular descriptive tool and take the consequences that follow.

> And consequences will indeed follow from that choice. The therapist's decision as to what the system "is" may very well determine the outcome of

therapy. Again, however, one must remember that if punctuating or describing the system this way "works" (i.e., facilitates successful intervention), all we can say is that it works, that it was useful. The fact that it works does not mean that it is accurate or truthful; it only means that it works. (16)

The concept of cooperating is more useful for a therapy based on an ecosystemic epistemology and the binocular theory of change than the concept of resistance would be. The particular behaviors, previously defined as resistance are now defined as cooperating. These behaviors are now described as a product of the interactional situation not as some property of the family subsystem.

The relationship between the concept of resistance and the concept of cooperating might be seen as two sides of the same coin. However, this is a restrictive view that creates imaginary oppositions. If a therapist chooses to see the family system's resistance, then the system's attempts to cooperate cannot be seen since each view precludes the other. If a therapist is looking for cooperating, then he will be unable to see the resistance. That is, both points of view — both types of descriptive tools — are initially attempting to describe different aspects of the same behaviors. The cooperating concept, based on the binocular theory of change, codes the information differently. Therefore, following the systemic principle of wholism, the use of the concept of cooperating will also effect the rest of the conceptual scheme (a system) because it is attuned to the processes of therapy over time.

Every part of a system is so related to its fellow parts that a change in one part will cause a change in all of them and in the total system. That is, a system behaves not as a simple composite of independent elements, but coherently as an inseparable whole. (62, p. 123)

The binocular theory of change, with its concurrent concepts of isomorphism and cooperating, suggests a model of therapy that is *not* a contest since the model excludes the concept of resistance.* Taken together, the two concepts can serve to guide the therapy team in describing the ecosystemic patterns and then in basing their interventions on this description. Using the con-

*From the earliest days, 20th-century psychotherapy has most often been described as a contest. In general, this contest was described as between the "forces" for change and the "forces" against change. The contest was this: The therapist (for change) had joined battle against the client's resistance (a force against change). Once the therapist "won" this contest, the client was no longer seen as resistant, and there was a "cure"; the problem was solved.

It seems unfortunate that much of psychotherapy and brief therapy (based on the concept of resistance) is frequently thought about and described in military and/or contest terms (34, 38, 52, 64). Therefore, a therapist is seen to plan strategy and then to implement tactics designed to deal with the family's resistance to change, and thus to promote change. In large part this is due to the concept of resistance itself, and in part this is due to the influence of Haley's (34) emphasis on the problem of control in therapy.

Haley's model (34, 40) is based largely on the old epistemology that included the concepts of power and control. His model developed logically from that foundation and from his early work with families that included a person diagnosed as "schizophrenic." To help a person change is par-

cept of isomorphism, the team can design reframing messages from a different angle that can promote the bonus of "extra depth" that can lead to change. Using the concept of cooperating, the therapy team can design tasks that promote behavior change that is isomorphic with the subsystem's patterns, but at a different angle—which further contributes to the bonus of extra depth. That is, the reframing gets directly at the meanings, or the cognitive aspects of the family system, which paves the way for change in behavior (since meaning and behavior belong to the same system). The tasks, or prescriptions, get directly at the behavior part of the system, which paves the way for change in the cognitive aspects of the system. (The task must also be isomorphic, but at an angle.) This means that the compliment and the clue (i.e., the reframing and the task) need to be isomorphic, which gives the intervention more "depth" because of the relationship between the two concepts as they are implemented.

Using the concurrent concepts of cooperating and isomorphism, the therapist is able to generate interventions that are fully accepting of the family's situation (although from a different angle), because we learned from Erickson that *any* response to any task that the family reports can be described as defining the family's unique way of attempting to cooperate. The task report is part of how they show this manner to the therapist. A positive, a negative, and an absence of response are all defined as responsive behavior.

> Any of the possibilities constitute responsive behavior. Thus a situation is created in which the subject can express his resistance in a constructive, cooperative fashion; manifestation of resistance by a subject is best utilized by developing a situation in which resistance serves a purpose. (35, p. 20)

Although Erickson uses the term "resistance," the term "cooperating" can be read in its place, and the behaviors can be seen as "manifestations of cooper-

---

ticularly difficult when he is as confused as a schizophrenic. In this light, it was a contest that needed power and control on the therapist's side because of the slippery and vague world view of the schizophrenic and his family. The problem of *who* is going to control *what* is central to *this situation*. Furthermore, Haley generalized the need for power and control to all therapy situations (38, 40). Again, this view of therapy can be seen to be based on the epistemological error of splitting the ecosystem and therefore creating imaginary oppositions. Certainly the family system of the schizophrenic and his family if described in terms of the closed, homeostatic system needs powerful techniques to induce change. (It should be noted here the Haley's techniques restated without the concepts of power and control can be ecosystemically useful in promoting change.)

Although the brief therapists at MRI do not use the concept of power or the concept of control as Haley does, their "judo-like techniques" (64) are also a metaphor from a contest. Like Haley, they see therapy as a contest between change and resistance to change. (Again, MRI's techniques can be restated to fit an ecosystemic model.) Both Haley's and MRI's work are part of the historical and contextual basis for this model of brief family therapy. This model suggests that no therapy need be seen as a contest, and the ecosystemic view—including the concept of cooperating—ends the need for contest terms.

ating." At the beginning of each session after the first, the conductor of the session (the member of the team in the room with the family) will elicit the family's responses to the previous session's tasks or clues. This will give the team information about the family's unique way of attempting to cooperate, regardless of the type of response the family reports. Thus, the definition of the family's unique manner of cooperating as shown to the team is further refined by the new knowledge gained in each session. The manner of cooperating as shown to the team can then further help the team refine or redefine their descriptions so that the reframing and the tasks can become more and more isomorphic.

PARADOX

Soper and L'Abate (58) and Dell (17) have suggested that part of the difficulty therapists have in understanding the nature of paradoxical intervention is because of a lack of a comprehensive theory. The binocular theory of change (with the concurrent concepts of isomorphism and cooperating) allows for a way of conceptualizing paradoxical interventions as part of a larger, more comprehensive theory than was available before. Central to this rethinking is that paradoxical interventions can be seen as "members" of a class of "isomorphic interventions" rather than being considered in a class by themselves. This way of looking at paradoxical interventions reemphasizes the counter double-bind nature of this technique and gives paradoxical interventions an ecosystemic basis with a theoretical frame. This construction allows a therapist to decide—based on suprasystemic information—when a paradoxical intervention is appropriate.

The deliberate use of "paradoxical interventions" or symptom prescriptions seems to go back to Dunlap's "negative practice" (25), although he did not call this method paradoxical. Frankl (29, 30) seems to have been the first to use the label "paradoxical." Haley (32) described the use of paradoxical techniques in trance inductions, and Jackson (46) wrote about the use of paradox with paranoid patients. Subsequently, many other therapists have described the use of paradoxical interventions mainly built on a model described by MRI (62, 64). The growth of interventions described as paradoxical has been rapid and extensive. This development has been catalogued, and the types of paradoxical interventions have been classified (58, 68, 69) and, therefore, will not be gone into here.

The MRI model is based on Russell's Theory of Types: *"Whatever involves all of a collection must not be one of the collection"* (62, p. 192). The model presupposes an intense relationship such as the family that includes a message described in such a way that

> (a) It asserts something, (b) it asserts something about its own assertion, and (c) these two assertions are mutually exclusive. Thus, if the message is an injunction, it must be disobeyed to be obeyed; if it is a definition of the self or the other, the person thereby defined is the kind of person only if he is not, and is not if he is. The meaning of the message is, therefore, undecidable. (62, p. 212)

Furthermore, the "recipient" of the message cannot effectively comment on it or withdraw from the relationship.

The Theory of Types has played a central role in the development of family therapy and brief therapy ever since the double-bind theory in "Toward a Theory of Schizophrenia"(5). * Not only did this paper (and subsequent papers by members of this group) influence how therapists *see* and *describe* families, it also influenced how therapists *treat* families. "Toward a Theory" proposed "a new way of conceptualizing and observing old problems," but it was "not so much a specific theory as a *language*—which like any language serves to orient both thinking and observing" (66, pp. 275-276).

> This language can be used to describe the family situation in which communication . . . becomes more and more cryptic in the mutual attempt to avoid exposure. They learn how to skillfully avoid any *patent* contradiction and become expert in the use of paradox, taking advantage of that possibility specific to man, to communicate simultaneously on the verbal and the non-verbal level, jumping from one logical class to a member of that class, as if they were the same thing, thus becoming acrobats in the world of Russellian paradox. (56, p. 25)

Not only can the language be used to describe the family's interaction, but it can also be used to describe interventions. In general, paradoxical interventions are seen as "curative factors . . . it is difficult to imagine that symptomatic double binds can be broken by anything other than counter double binds" (62, p. 240). Thus the treatment of "pathogenic" double binds is seen to involve counter double binds or paradoxical interventions. Structurally, a therapeutic double bind is the mirror image of a pathogenic one. First, the counter double bind presupposes an intense relationship that is highly valued by the client. Second,

> an injunction is given which is so constructed that it (a) reinforces the behavior the patient expects to be changed, (b) implies that this reinforcement is the vehicle of change, and (c) thereby creates paradox because the patient is told to change by remaining unchanged. (62, p. 241)

---

*The Theory of Types was an attempt to rid logic and mathematics of self-referential paradoxes. Spencer-Brown (60) resolved this problem and presented Russell "with the proof that it was unnecessary. To my relief he was delighted. The Theory, he said, was the most arbitrary thing he and Whitehead had ever had to do, not really a theory but a stopgap, and he was glad to have lived long enough to see the matter resolved" (60, p. xiv). However, the Theory remains viable as a descriptive tool.

Third, the therapeutic situation is described as preventing the patient from withdrawing and/or effectively commenting on the paradox.

The idea behind this is to *break* the symptomatic double bind with a counter double bind. This notion is congruent with Russell's Theory of Types: namely, that self-referential statements need to be eliminated from logic. Among others, Hofstadter (43) and Spencer-Brown (60) have described the arbitrary and unnecessary nature of the Theory of Types. Furthermore, the use of the Theory in the field of family therapy seems to have restricted our thinking and hindered the development of ecosystemic descriptions of the observed phenomena. As an example of this, the fascination with paradox (and counter-paradox) has sometimes led to a bit of a muddle in the field of family therapy and family therapy research, a result of the frequent "misunderstanding of the double-bind theory" that Watzlawick explores (63).

Using the binocular theory of change, paradoxical interventions can be seen as just one form of isomorphic intervention that a therapist can design and give to a family. It is important to recognize that the paradoxical intervention is a *counter* double bind, a mirror image, which is appropriate to the structure of the family's *pathogenic* double bind. When a therapist's description of the family patterns does *not* include a double bind, then his intervention needs to follow the family's patterns in some other manner that is isomorphic with the family's patterns. The intervention needs to *fit* the observed patterns isomorphically, which the counter-double-bind pattern does when it mirrors the family's pathogenic double bind.

In either case, with or without a paradox, the intervention needs to be isomorphic with the family patterns, and the intervention needs to be presented from a different angle so that the family can get the desired bonus.

Furthermore, this fascination with "paradox" and "paradoxical interventions" also stems from the therapists' use of what is commonly called "reverse psychology." That is, the therapist tells the client to do something deliberately in order to stop the client from doing it. This procedure is often (mis)labeled "paradoxing":

> But, can an event be paradoxical if it is expected? This question is central to the whole concept of paradox in therapy. Remember again, that to operate from consistent but invalid premises tends to yield an unexpected and paradoxical outcome. (17, p. 41)

The therapist operating from an ecosystemic or interactional point of view fully expects the procedure of "reverse psychology" to stop the symptom. Now the client or an observer may view this outcome as a surprise. However, he can be seen to be viewing this outcome from another perspective built on Aristotelian premises, and, therefore, given this framework, he is surprised because these premises are systemically invalid (17). The outcome appears absurd or even magical. The conclusion sounds absurd, and the reverse psychology is the only argument to sustain it; therefore, the intervention is mislabeled as paradoxical.

The binocular theory construction can help to clear up some misunderstanding of paradoxical interventions so that some conceptual muddles can be avoided. A lot of research strategies have been developed to test the effects of paradox and paradoxical interventions. However, these have usually been inconclusive. What seems to happen most frequently is that the researchers reify the double bind or the paradox. That is, what they seem to do is use one element of a systemic or interactional concept in a lineal fashion, thus removing the paradox and the paradoxical intervention from its context. Because of the lack of a clear, comprehensive theory, they seemed not to recognize that paradoxical interventions are part of a *pattern* of matching the (paradoxical) intervention isomorphically with the family's (paradoxical) pattern. These researchers and therapists used the reified paradox in a linear (cause-effect) manner to attempt to study and promote change. Thus, they seem to view the thing "paradox" as the agent of change, and therefore they will paradox clients, rather than seeing the *fit* between the intervention pattern and the family pattern as the key to promoting change. This later view has been implicit since "Toward a Theory" (5) and has become more (6) and more explicit (56) leading up to the development of the binocular theory that incorporates paradoxical interventions as counterparadoxes within the larger class of isomorphic interventions.

The reasoning to which we have restricted ourselves (because of the Theory of Types and because of the perception of paradoxical interventions as a class) has limited our perception of a useful therapeutic approach. The binocular theory of change suggests that isomorphic reframing messages can be useful regardless of the "type" of family patterns observed and codified. Paradoxical interventions can then be seen as one type of isomorphic intervention, and therefore the therapist can use this particular type of intervention appropriately when the patterns he observes are described as paradoxical. However, when the patterns he observes are *not* described as paradoxical, the isomorphic intervention will follow a different map because the territory is different. This way of thinking can help the field of family therapy become less restricted in conceptualizing and can help the development of progressively more useful ecosystemic concepts that will lead to solving some problems of research conceptualization and methodology.

CHAPTER 2

The Clinical Context

There is a complex relationship among theoretical developments, clinical practice, clinical research, and the culture or context in which these endeavors occur. The binocular theory of change and the brief family therapy model are not exceptions. Their growth and development are based on roots or foundations found in the works of other therapists.

A WORLD VIEW

Many different ways exist to conceptualize the tasks of the brief family therapist. Each of these ways is an imprecise, even metaphorical, description of the therapist's world view. This world view allows therapists to construct their experiences with clients in a manner that makes the family's world view and its experiences at least partially comprehensible to the therapists. Otherwise, other people's problems and puzzles might seem beyond understanding. At first glance, any "troublesome behavior" can appear rather strange. It would seem reasonable for a person troubled by a certain behavior simply to stop that behavior. But, as we all know, breaking any habit is not easy, particularly when we think we must, or others insist we must.

To illustrate, Milton Erickson describes a young man who could urinate only through an 8- to 10-inch-long wooden or iron pipe held at the end of his penis. As unreasonable and strange as this behavior was, it made sense to the young man. Erickson understood this. Therefore, he taught the young man to urinate through a 12-inch bamboo tube. In Erickson's view, if he could first lengthen the tube and change the material, then (by implication) he could also shorten it. Erickson knew better than to try talking the young man into giving up the pipe. Undoubtedly, he had tried talking himself out of this behavior, and Erickson did not join him in this unsuccessful effort. The young man knew he was strange, and that the tube was unreasonable, but this knowledge had not stopped him from using the pipe. In response to Erickson's suggestions, over the next three months, the young man was able to shorten the tube until the remaining "tube" held by his fingers was his penis.

When this therapy was performed, most other therapists would have seen Erickson's approach as unreasonable and strange, as unreasonable and as strange as the young man's behavior. According to contemporary standards, Erickson should have delved into the unconscious reasons "why" the young man thought the pipe was necessary. Once this why was understood, the young man could have stopped the troublesome behavior. This process, which might be called "standard psychotherapy," might have been just as effective, though it could have taken a lot longer than three months. Apparently, Erickson's therapy is based on a different set of premises.

Erickson's world view makes therapy "predicated upon the assumption that there is a strong tendency for the personality to adjust if given the opportunity" (35, p. 417). This procedure was designed to give the young man exactly that opportunity. Furthermore, Erickson's method was quick. While the young man was in a deep trance, the suggestions for the next three months were given to him. Thus the problem could be seen as solved by the young man himself. When the young man saw Erickson again, the problem was solved.

By the 1980s Erickson's treatment of this case (first published in 1954) no longer seemed quite so strange and unreasonable. This is not to say that this procedure (and the epistemology behind it) serves as a prototype of contemporary standard psychotherapy. Rather, this method is no longer so unique that it appears idiosyncratic: the work of a genius, magician, or wizard. Therapy that follows this prototype is the work of only a minority of psychotherapists. However, it is a product of a world view that is growing in acceptance within the therapeutic community.

A large measure of this growing acceptance is the result of work by a group of therapists who have attempted to explain Erickson's world view and methods to the therapeutic professions. Haley (34, 35, 37) aimed to explain Erickson's methods and to expand the principles into a comprehensive model of "strategic therapy." Over the years the work of the members of the MRI (Jackson, Weakland, Watzlawick, Fisch, and, in the early years, Haley) has been based on the developments that have grown out of their understanding of Erickson's work (62, 64, 67). From this base, first, they contributed to the development of family therapy and, then, to brief therapy, based on the same world view. While Haley and MRI concentrated on the central, underlying principles, Bandler and Grinder (2, 3) developed guidelines for the use of some of Erickson's techniques.

Of course, none of these authors either separately or in combination have mined all the ore in the Erickson lode. Each of these authors, and others including de Shazer (18, 20, 21, 23), has attempted to describe the effective methods of change Erickson developed. de Shazer (21) developed a model of change based on Erickson's work as understood through the use of Heider's balance theory (41). From this basic model (see Chapter 6), different therapy situations can be mapped out and described in a goal-directed manner. In the years of trying to solve problems in an Ericksonian manner, certain tools have developed for understanding and mapping out problems that people found "insolvable" enough to bring to therapy. Simply, the therapist's world view must help him to see beyond the client's world view. The therapist must see the client's problem from a different angle.

> A Japanese coastal village was once threatened by a tidal wave but the wave was sighted in advance, far out on the horizon, by a lone farmer in the rice fields on the hillside above the village. At once he set fire to the fields, and the villagers who came swarming up to save their crops were saved from the flood. (61, p. 71)

This lone farmer had a puzzle to solve: how to save the villagers from the flood? Probably he was too far from the village to yell a warning and knew he did not have time to run down to the village to evacuate everybody. The problem seems insolvable. But in the resolution found by the lone farmer a world view similar to Erickson's can be seen at work. The lone farmer (seeing the problem from a different angle) deceived the villagers into solving the fire problem that accidentally solved the flood problem. He knew that setting the fire would attract the villagers' attention. Thus, they were able "spontaneously" to save themselves from the flood. Although the villagers were probably thankful to the lone farmer for saving them from the flood, they were also probably angry at him for burning the rice crop. Crops grow again, but individual people do not.

Their attitude might have been similar to that of one of Erickson's former patients who

> never fails to send me a Christmas card, but he always writes: "I hate your guts and I'm going to keep right on." Nevertheless, he sends Christmas presents to my children, but he always has a nasty crack for me. When we meet, we laugh and talk and exchange stories. . . . "But," he has told me, "it seems to me I've got a lifelong hatred of something—I don't know what it is. You're convenient, and you're a nice guy to hate."
> I said, "That's right, and it's solved your stammering problem." (26, p.33)

Resolving a puzzle described from a different angle that is designed to solve the original problem is a feature common to Erickson's work and the work of various other brief therapists. Like the Japanese villagers, it is probably not important for families to know that they are solving one problem that can accidentally and spontaneously solve another problem. It can be imagined that the villagers became aware of the reason for the deception once they saw their village flooded. Some families become aware that the changes they have made helped them reach the goals they have had for therapy. Others do not; they realize they have reached their goal but do not connect it with the changes they have made in therapy.

It is very important for therapists not to attempt to solve the family's puzzles by doing what it is already doing. The therapists, at least, must see the puzzle from a different angle. If Erickson had tried to talk the young man out of using the pipe, the problem might have escalated, and the young man might still be using the pipe.

Of course, not all problems are similar to the young man's or the Japanese villager's. Different contexts develop different problems, and the therapy needs to be different. Whatever the problem pattern and whatever the therapeutic procedure, each therapy situation needs to include a "specific goal." For the lone farmer, the goal was to save the villagers from the flood. For the young man, the goal was to urinate in a normal fashion. In each situation, the *reframing* (seeing a puzzle from a different angle) allowed the goal to be achieved. The original frame (or angle) had prevented solution.

FRAMES

It is easy to agree with Dorothy Sayers' Lord Peter Wimsey that "life is just one damn thing after another." What people do with those damn things seems to vary widely. Some of what people do seems to work well, and life goes on with moderate ups and downs. As therapists, we do not hear much about what people do that works well, but we do hear a lot about what does not work for a particular family in a particular context. We find this out when a family describes its futile attempts to eliminate the complaints that bring them to therapy.

If one is able to accept Lord Peter's definition, then life can flow along with its little ripples. Lord Peter thinks and operates in terms of this definition, which helps him to define situations in his life. Of course, this definition is only a part of a set of rules that we can infer from reading Dorothy Sayers' books. This set of infered rules is used to "frame" situations (i.e., to define what it is that is going on). Similarly, Erickson's notion, that if given the opportunity, people will adjust, is part of the set of rules he used to define what is is that is going on in the therapy situation.

Both Bateson (7) and Goffman (31) defined "frames" in ways that are useful in understanding the complaints people bring to therapy. Goffman states that people's "definitions of a situation are built up in accordance with principles of organization which govern events—at least social ones—and our subjective involvement in them" (31, p.10). A frame can be compared with the rules of a game, or with a " 'code' as a device which informs and patterns all events that fall within the boundaries of its application" (31, p.7). Frames, in short, operate as if they are the rules that define situations.

The family thinks and operates as though it has a certain set of rules or overlapping sets of individual rules plus "unit rules," which are used to define its situation. For instance, these definitions could be seen to include "what is serious versus what is not serious," "what is good versus what is not good," and "how to show love versus how not to show love." These are only samples of the types of inferred definitions that can be included in a description of a family's frame. Obviously, many more rules (inferred by the observer) are necessary to have a full description of a family's frames.

It is easy to see how two individuals coming from different families can quickly get into conflict. For example, if one individual is from a family with a Germanic heritage, various sausages and meats will form a large part of what is "the proper way to eat." If another individual is from Japan with a strong Buddhist background, then not eating meat is "the proper way to eat." If, in spite of these differences these two find enough in their world views that is similar, they might become friends and even marry and start a new family. But what about the conflictual rules about the proper way to eat? Various options exist, including separate meals. But most likely there will be some conflict and one or the other rule* will change. Or both. And the proper way to eat will have a new definition. Usually most couples' differing frames will be more subtle than "meat versus nonmeat." Neither of the individuals is necessarily aware that these differences in rules, definitions, and frames exist: The terms "rules," "definitions," and "frames" are only descriptive tools of an observer. But frames define situations and people's subjective involvement in these situations. For example, a couple's unspoken frames might have different rules about which behaviors can be included in "how to show love versus how not to show love."

It is these differences in frames that seem common to many of the complaints families bring to therapists. The individuals will not talk about frames, but they will describe unacceptable behaviors that the other person thinks quite acceptable, reasonable, and "normal." For instance, the range of behaviors that might be included in the "ways to show love" might be very narrow, and therefore, the range of behaviors of "ways not to show love" might be correspondingly large. People usually do not see the other person's behavior as being part of their "in" frame, but rather they see the other person's behavior as part of their own "out" frame.

This "in versus out" or "on versus off" nature of definitions and frames is somewhat similar to the way a thermostat works, except that human systems operate without an "outsider" determining the settings. Under most situations when we set a thermostat at 65 degrees, the furnace will click on at the bottom of a range of temperatures and off at the top of that range. In principle, the temperature should hover around the 65-degree mark without wild variations.

---

* It must be remembered that this means that people behave "as if" there are rules. The attribution of "rules" is part of the observer's effort to define what it is that is going on.

However, if the range of acceptable temperatures is too narrow, then the furnace will go off/on/off in a wild, confused pattern. The thermostat will be unable to determine which setting is on when the range is too narrow.

Jackson (44) observed redundant or recurring patterns of behavior in families and suggested that these patterns could be understood as following rules. At the beginning, Jackson seemed to suggest that these rules provided the reason for the redundancy of the observed patterns. These rules were generally understood to be "homeostatic mechanisms" that regulated what happens between the family members (44). Subsequently, Jackson clarified this and described these rules as an "as if" description by the observer for the purpose of conceptualizing what it is that is going on.

Since families can be seen to operate as if there are certain sets of rules (62) and these rules define how they perceive a situation, the possibilities for confusion and conflict abound. It is this "one damn thing after another" that makes up the everyday difficulties (64) with which people need to deal. And if they accept that part of Lord Peter's frame, then events can flow on in irregular patterns; but this rule is often not part of people's frames. Most people tend to see these difficulties as "something to be corrected" and the "problem" (64) develops when this attempted solution fails.

For example, children will sometimes wet their bed, men will sometimes ejaculate prematurely, and women will sometimes not have orgasms. Each of these qualify as "one of those damn things." But if people attempt to "solve" these "things" as though they are problems, the attempted solution might not work (most do not) and another attempt is called for. Now there are *two* problems: the event itself and the failed solution. A bigger problem ensues because the correction (attempted solution) seemed the only logical thing to do. Since it failed, Western logic calls for another attempt that must be bigger and better. But that usually does not work either. The person is trapped into doing "more of the same" (64) of something that did not work.

REFRAMING

There are certain similarities between people's frames and the rules of a game that serve to define the nature of the game itself and to proscribe and prescribe certain behaviors. For instance, if two canasta players play for the first time together, they might each assume that the other knows the rules. Therefore, the game will go along just fine. One will lose, the other will win, both of which are part of the game. However, there are local variations in canasta rules that have been informally determined. If, in the middle of the game one player follows a local custom that violates the formal rules of the game, the two players can stop and discuss this violation. They can decide which rule to follow, and the game will go on.

But in relationships each individual considers the frame he uses (local custom) to be the formal rules of the game. When another individual violates that frame or that part of the frame, the violator can be seen as bad, crazy, or just wrong. Of course, the "violator" sees his behavior as following the formal rules of the game, thus seeing the other as mistaken (at best). But, there are no formal rules of the "relationship game," and the groundwork is set for making a problem of a difficulty.

According to Bateson, an individual "after successful therapy operates in terms of a different set of such rules" (7, p. 191) that make up his frame. The same can be said for successful therapy with a family: The family operates in terms of a different set, or sets, of such rules that make up its frame.

"Brief family therapy" can be described as an attempt to help people change the frames that cause them trouble and give them reason to complain. In general, the therapy is designed to change the definitions that make up a family's frame and to do this in a gradual fashion. This process of changing frames is called "reframing," which means

> to change the conceptual and/or emotional setting or viewpoint in relation to which a situation is experienced and to place it in another frame which fits the "facts" of the same concrete situation equally well or even better, and thereby changes its entire meaning. (64, p. 95)

Although the "facts" of the situation are not changed, the context in which they lie is described by the therapist from a different angle, and therefore the intervention (or reframing) is in positive terms rather than in the negative terms used by the family. The effects of reframing are confirmed by the appearance of a new set of beliefs, or perceptions, and behavioral modifications that can be described as a logical consequence of the shift in perception. Most frequently the family's new frames are combinations of the old frame and the suggested new frames offered by the therapist. The result is that the family can look at things from a different angle. Once they "see things differently," they can behave differently.

The binocular theory of change is built around the difference that reframing creates. The original frame (A), together with the new frame (A_1), starts the change process because it changes the family's perception of its situation. This allows for new behavior that in turn allows for the creation of new subjective experiences.

Most families seem to accept changes in their frames slowly and cautiously. It is as if they can accept a change in definition only if one word at a time is allowed to change. After successful therapy, the family can be seen to have a new set of rules and definitions—new frames. The range of acceptable behaviors might be widened or narrowed if needed. More events can then be seen as one of those "damn things" that constitute life. The family is more able to accept Lord Peter's definition.

Therapists as well as clients can be seen to use frames to help them define situations. Two new behaviors helped the BFTC redefine or reframe the therapy situation for themselves: the "consulting break" and the "compliment." Both of these activities helped to change the perception of the therapy situation to a view that lead to a change in the therapy frame. Since frames are part of conceptual systems, these changes in behavior also had some profound effects on the rest of the conceptual model that developed from the work of Milton Erickson and the MRI.

MILTON H. ERICKSON

Milton H. Erickson, M.D., is generally acknowledged to be the world's leading practioner of medical hypnosis. His writings on hypnosis are the authoritative word on techniques of inducing trance, experimental work exploring the possibilities and limits of inducing trance, and investigations of the nature of the relationship between hypnotist and subject. (35, p. 1)

Brief family therapy owes a large debt to Milton Erickson's methods of therapy and the world view that these imply. His procedures involve a "process of evoking and utilizing a patient's own mental process in ways that are outside his usual range of intentional or voluntary control" (28, p. 19). Erickson takes the learnings people already have and helps them to apply these in other ways. That is, Erickson can be seen to accept the person's world view and the patterns in which the person is involved; then he helps the person use these patterns in new ways. Erickson is rightly "wary about suggesting or adding anything new to the patient: he would rather facilitate the patient's ability to creatively utilize and develop what he already has" (28, p. 5). This way of thinking led Erickson to develop a wide variety of approaches to human problems because his approach is built on the unique world views and patterns of the patient.

At one extreme, Erickson may talk roughly to a man helpless in a chair, calling him typical of the "God damn Nazis!" in hopes of motivating the man through anger or pride. At the other extreme, he may talk softly and patiently to Joe, an old florist, using a metaphor about tomato plants to help Joe subtly deal with the pains of terminal cancer (37).

The therapist wishing to help his patient should never scorn, condemn nor reject any part of a patient's conduct simply because it is obstructive, unreasonable or even irrational. . . . The therapist should not limit himself to an appraisal of what is good and reasonable as offering possible foundations for therapeutic procedures. Sometimes, in fact, many more times than is realized, therapy can be firmly established on a sound basis only by the utilization of silly, absurd, irrational, and contradictory manifestations. (35, p. 500)

Erickson's knowledge of and acceptance of the wide variety of human patterns led him to a wide range of ways he implements his therapeutic designs. His sage-like wisdom and creativity made these methods appear idiosyncratic and gimmicky. Erickson's books (27, 28) and his many papers (35, 37) detail the scope of his methods without developing a comprehensive theory or model of therapy.

In fact, these methods may appear so unique and so outside the standard practice of psychotherapy and hypnotherapy that each seems a stroke of genius well beyond the talents of most other therapists. As Haley states:

> It is this wide variety which makes his therapeutic approach difficult to encapsulate in some general theory of therapy. Obviously, there are basic principles on which he operates: one can recognize an Erickson therapeutic procedure as easily as a Picasso painting. (35, p. 534)

As Erickson himself said, "I know what I do, but to explain how I do it is much too difficult for me" (2, p. viii). The number of explanations available seems to match the wide variety of Erickson's methods, and perhaps all of these are correct when taken as a whole.

These principles have long been evident in Erickson's work:

1. Meet the patient where he is at, and gain rapport.
2. Modify the patient's productions and gain control.
3. Use the control that has been established to structure the situation so that change, when it does occur, will occur in a desirable manner and a manner compatible with the patient's inner wishes and inner drive. (10, p. 59)

For example, a man came to Erickson for hypnosis. The man paced around the office seemingly unwilling and unable to sit down. Erickson asked, " 'Are you willing to cooperate with me by continuing to pace the floor, even as you are now doing?' His reply was a startled, 'Willing? Good God, man! I've got to do it if I stay in the office' " (35, p. 34). Erickson met the patient where he was and gained rapport. Thus Erickson was able to set the foundation for therapy by directing, at least in part, the man's pacing behavior since the pacing was now *responsive* rather than *obstructive*. The man's pattern (at that moment) included pacing, and Erickson cooperated with the man's way by telling him to pace. Then, when the man responded by continuing to pace, Erickson could modify the behavior by telling the man where in the office to pace, thus gaining control. This utilization technique "meets both the patient's presenting needs and it employs as the significant part of the induction procedure the very behavior that dominates the patient" (35, p. 35).

The brief family therapy model is designed to make the principles behind Erickson's methods explicit enough for other therapists without Erickson's particular gifts. The model expands these principles from the field of hypnotherapy to the field of family therapy. The model is designed to be concise enough so that other therapists can find its use effective, which allows us to agree with Mara Selvini-Palazzoli "that success in therapy is not dependent upon the charismatic personality of . . . the therapists, but rather upon the method followed. In truth, *if the method is correct, no charisma whatsoever is needed*" (56, p. 11). Although Erickson looms charismatically large in the background, the methods are effective without the charisma. It was through BFTC's efforts to apply Erickson's methods and procedures that our approach was developed, and the binocular theory of change owes a lot to that process.

THE MENTAL RESEARCH INSTITUTE

The brief therapy group at MRI (64, 67) also has part of their roots in Milton Erickson. They have developed an approach to therapy that views clients' problems as aspects of ongoing interaction. Their model is based on their earlier work (5, 62), which conceptualized the family and therapy through the lens of Russellian paradox. They describe "disturbed, deviant, or difficult behavior in an individual (like behavior generally) as essentially a social phenomenon, occurring as one aspect of a system, reflecting some dysfunction in that system, and best treated by some appropriate modification of that system" (67, p. 145). Their focus is explicitly "pragmatic," and they focus on practical approaches to human problem solving designed to be as economical and as simple as possible.

In keeping with this focus, the group is very goal directed, and they value tools and techniques on the basis of their utility in reaching goals. Many of these techniques, and the principles behind these techniques, are derived from the work of Milton Erickson, although their "conceptualization of problems and treatment appears at least more general and explicit than Erickson's and probably [is] different in various specific respects" (67, p. 146).

What is strikingly distinctive about this group is its emphasis on the nature of problem formation and problem solution. Basically, its view describes problems as the result of mishandling of everyday events, which then are maintained by the very efforts people make to resolve this situation.

> Consider, for instance, a common pattern between a depressed patient and his family. The more they try to cheer him up and make him see the positive sides of life, the more depressed the patient is likely to get: "They don't even understand me." The action meant to *alleviate* the behavior of the other party aggravates it; the "cure" becomes worse than the original disease."
> (67, p. 149)

Brief therapy, then, is designed to interrupt this pattern and to substitute a new pattern of behavior. For instance, the MRI group might help the depressed person's family stop aggravating the situation by stopping the family's efforts "to cheer him up" (60). In turn, this "stopping of the cure" can help the depressed person become less depressed or even help him stop being depressed.

> We contend generally that change can be effected most easily if the goal of change is reasonably small and clearly stated. Once the patient has experienced a small but definite change in the seemingly monolithic nature of the problem most real to him, the experience leads to further, self-induced changes in this, and often also, in other areas of his life. (67, p. 150)

The very strength of the MRI model, which is that it is pragmatic and goal directed is also the main weakness. Nowhere (15, 64, 65, 67) does the group explicitly deal with the brief therapy approach used with people who have mutually exclusive goals or with people who have vague, ill-formed goals that they are unable to articulate. This limitation in the scope of the MRI brief therapy model led de Shazer to attempt to expand the model to deal with mutually exclusive goals (18). Although the original expansion of the scope of MRI's was intended as simply that, subsequent chapters will show the new brief family therapy model that developed in large part from that initial effort.

THE MILAN GROUP

From the same roots (5, 62) another model of brief therapy developed in Milan (55, 56). Although influenced by the brief therapists of MRI (in particular, the yearly visits of Watzlawick), this group's work is mostly derived from Watzlawick's earlier work (62) and Haley's model of the schizophrenic family (33).

> This work offered us the proper instruments for the analysis of communication: the concept of context as matrix of meanings; the notion of the coexistence of two languages, the analogic and the digital; the concept of punctuation in interaction, the concept of the necessity to define the relationship and the various verbal and nonverbal levels which can be used to define it; the notion of symmetrical and complementary positions in relationships; and the fundamental notion of symptomatic and therapeutic paradox. (56, p. 8)

A major contribution of this group is the notion of "positive connotation" (56), which developed out of the therapist's need to avoid contradicting himself should he, later in the session, choose to use a counterparadox and prescribe the symptom. However, just positively connoting the identified patient's symptom is not systemic, and the Milan group makes great efforts to be consistently systemic. Therefore, the group will positively connote not only the symptom but the patterns that surround that symptom.

In other words, by qualifying "symptomatic" behaviors as "positive" or "good" because they are motivated by the homeostatic tendency, *what we are connoting positively is the homeostatic tendency of the system, and not its members.* (56, p. 58)

The Milan group is also very conscious of the difficulty in thinking systemically or circularly because Occidental language is linear by nature. "Since rational thought is formed through language, we conceptualize reality (whatever that may be) according to the linguistic model which thus becomes for us the same thing as reality" (56, p. 52). As an aid to stepping outside this trap, the group suggests that therapists substitute the verb "to seem" for the verb "to be." As a next step, it further suggests a substitution of the verb "to show" for the verb "to seem." According to the Milan group, this step in the description helps to make the game-like events stand out clearly. Therefore, it describes therapy as similar to a chess game in which little or nothing is known about the opponents except *how* they play. This is clear from the title of the Milan group's book, *Paradox and Counterparadox,* which shows that it understands that a counter double bind is only useful in a situation (or game) that involves a double bind.

Since the Milan group's theory of change is based on the concept of homeostasis, it creates epistemologically false "imaginary oppositions" that lead it to see therapy as a contest or "game." That is, it views the situation as "counterparadox versus paradox." This is extremely curious since its format, like BFTC's, includes a break in the session that is used for the team to design interventions. Its interventions are generally phrased as coming from the group as a whole in order to strengthen the power of the therapist in the game against the power of the family system's homeostatic resistance to change. Although the group behaves as if it has broken through the mirror as a shield, nonetheless it continues to see the family as "out there" and as a subject for study by detached observers.

CHAPTER 3

Procedures

"I could never do that. Although these methods seem to work, it is sort of like magic. Even if I could think of the intervention, I could never convince my clients to do the tasks."

Variations of this remark have been heard by every brief therapist, strategic therapist, or brief family therapist who has explained or demonstrated his approach to other, more traditional, therapists. The procedures used at BFTC have been developed, at least in part, as a teaching method in response to this type of remark. As long as the therapist uses the concept of resistance and Aristotelian premises, designing interventions remains difficult to explain. Ecosystemic premises and the binocular theory of change make it easier to design interventions and to teach the designing skills.

Another important aspect of the procedures is that BFTC is very interested in the fit between theory and practice. Therefore, the interventions are very carefully designed, and the effects on the family system from session to session are studied by the part of the team behind the mirror. From one session to the next the team attempts to predict the response that the family will report following an intervention.

Describing and utilizing the family's manner of cooperating are other aspects of our ongoing study and of the experimental nature of BFTC's approach. When the conductor is delivering the compliment after the consulting break (and before giving the family a "clue" about solving its puzzle) the team carefully notes how the family shows its responses to the team's statements. From the reactions the family shows, the team has some indication of how successful it has been in its effort to describe (to itself) the family patterns in an isomorphic fashion. Also, from the responses the family shows to the compliment, the team will predict how the family will respond to the clue that is usually given in task form. From the reaction the family shows to both elements of the therapeutic message, the team predicts the type of response to the clue the family will report in the following session.

At BFTC the therapy session is divided into six sections: (1) presession planning, (2) the prelude, (3) data collecting, (4) the consulting break: intervention designing, (5) message giving: intervening, and (6) study efforts. The session lasts approximately one hour with the consulting break starting after the first 40 minutes. The same format is used in all sessions, although it can be modified as needed in later sessions. The activities will be described for both the conductor and the rest of the team behind the mirror. A different typeface will be used when describing the tasks behind the mirror.

The methods the team uses behind the mirror are meant to operationalize the concurrent concepts of isomorphism and cooperating. The team's task is not to develop a linear description of the family system or of the therapeutic interaction. Rather, its task is to describe the patterns the family describes and shows. Due to the limitations of the English language, the descriptions of circular data and the methods for collecting these data have to be presented in sequential fashion. However, the results are more circular than they are linear because of the mapping procedures. Of course the "map is not the territory," and, therefore, all descriptions are only approximate.

PRESESSION PLANNING

Prior to the first session the team compares notes about other cases in its experience that included some similar elements of the situation as described by the family member who made the appointment. If, for example, the family includes a bed wetter, the team will discuss previously noted patterns of interaction around this complaint and previously noted patterns of intervention that have been found effective in at least some similar situations. The team will develop a temporary guide to suggest to the conductor certain kinds of information which seemed pertinent with other families that included a bed wetter. This is done quickly and sketchily so as not to bias the conductor's efforts to collect meaningful data from a particular family.

(In general, the team will include therapists with different levels of experience. The team can include experienced brief family therapists, experienced family therapists, therapists trained in other models, postgraduate trainees, and graduate students. Since the number of people can be quite large, these differences help insure that the team will not let the conductor get stuck in looking for data from a too rigidly predetermined point of view. That is, these differences help prevent the team from getting locked into a temporary guide that may not prove helpful. The presence of more than one systemic or ecosystemic thinker behind the mirror often provides the team with different maps of the family and therapy systems. This increases the team's ability to achieve an isomorphic map.)

THE PRELUDE

(In musical terms, a preliminary part of a composition that serves as an introduction. A section or movement that introduces the themes, which is an integral part of the composition.)

During this phase of the session, usually about 10 minutes in length, the conductor avoids (when possible) all discussion of the complaints that brought the family to therapy. Instead, he focuses on the social context of the family. His questions center around where the family lives, what the neighborhood is like, what religion the family practices, what kind of work each person does, and what schools the children attend. Any area of life is explored sketchily as long as it does not seem connected with the complaints. In general, the conductor adopts a casual approach to gathering this information and sets a socializing, small talk mood. He is trying to build a nonthreatening, helpful relationship with the whole family and to learn something about how the family sees its world.

Behind the mirror, the team is watching the patterns the family shows. Will they follow the conductor's agenda and talk about these nonproblem areas, or will they push on directly to the complaints? The team will, for example, note who talks most and to whom, whether one person speaks for another, who is most silent, and the favorite phrases each person uses to describe something that is not a problem. It is important for the team to notice vocabulary and occupations since these may indicate, in part, the way the family sees the world and thus will allow the team to be more isomorphic in its description. (It is one thing to have a bed wetter when the family has a father who works third shift in a factory, another to have the same complaint in a family where the father is a minister, and yet another when the family is without a father.)

To a lesser extent the team notes the predicates each family member uses: (1) visual, auditory, kinesthetic, or (2) cognitive. This seems less important than the particular phrases each person uses, but it can be useful information if the team notices that the conductor is having trouble talking with one individual family member. Putting together the special phrases and the favorite words enhances the team's ability to communicate with a family and helps the team design interventions that are isomorphic. However, both of these seem secondary to matching the team's words with the family's world view and its patterns.

Some families and some individuals shift their favorite phrases and predicates when addressing a problem (i.e., they use different words to describe other aspects of their total situation). When this is the case, the team will note it and will use the nonproblem words (noted during the prelude) when designing and delivering the therapeutic message. This is done to help the family perceive the news of a difference and to thus promote change.

DATA COLLECTING

After about 10 minutes, the conductor shifts from the prelude to the main body of the session (approximately 30 to 35 minutes in length) by asking the family: "Well, what problem can *we* help you with?" This sort of question is usually asked of the family as a whole rather than of any individual. The *response* is sometimes an indicator of who is most bothered by the complaint. Sometimes the discussion about *who* is to answer can give the team information about how decisions are made and what the relationships among the people are like.

Once someone has responded, the conductor will elicit each individual's different view of the same information. Since each person perceives the situation differently, the conductor brings out this information to assist the team in its intervention designing task.

Throughout the session the conductor's attitude is as noncritical as possible, although this does not mean inactive. Everything the family says and does is accepted as "normal enough and natural enough *given the situation.*" In general, the conductor's comments are aimed at clarifying the descriptions. He will attempt to help the family be as specific as possible about its situation.

The conductor takes particular care to find out what the family has done to attempt to solve the puzzle it brought to therapy. (Are the family's attempts to deal with the problem actually serving to aggravate it?) For example, the family with a bed wetter may go the entire medical route to attempt a cure without ever considering the child as a "problem child." Or, they may consider bed wetting as naughty and therefore punish the child. Some families will take the child to church and pray for him; others may consider bed wetting to be normal, but their physician, pastor, or the school may be troubled by the situation. It is important to differentiate each of these variations on the bed-wetting theme. Each of these situations in different families will probably have very different patterns, and the families' ways of cooperating will be different.

By approving the family's efforts to deal with its complaints, the conductor is, of course, building his relationship with the family. He is also learning how the family members cooperate with other people and among themselves. By being noncritical, the conductor is also keeping the options open for the team to compliment the family about its efforts.

Getting the family members to talk with and about each other is helpful to the team's effort to collect pattern data. An indirect method seems much more effective than the direct way of telling the people to "talk to each other about this." For example, if the discussion has been around when the girl is aware of sucking her thumb and what the mother does to try and stop this behavior, the conductor can ask a third person for his observations of what happens between mother and daughter around this interaction; that is, father can be asked about what happens when mother sees daughter sucking her thumb. Mother can then be asked about what goes on when father catches the girl, and the girl can be asked what then happens between mother and father. It seems much easier for people to describe interactions between two other people than to describe interactions in which they play an active role. If there is a fourth person, for example, a brother, even more observation data can be obtained if he can describe what happens among the other three. Sometimes the views match, sometimes not. Either way these descriptions give the team some data about how the family members each perceive the other. Since people seem to like to correct each other, this "interactional interviewing technique" can often prompt some lively discussion among the family members that is relevant to the task. That is, in response to these types of questions, the family gives the team information about its "frames" and about the behavioral sequence.

In some situations the family members will describe a set of complaints that seem related to each other; in other situations they might describe problems that seem unrelated. It is the conductor's job to help them focus on one particular complaint on which to begin working. However, this sort of focus is not always possible. Frequently, the various complaints will follow the same pattern (or metapattern), and therefore the choice of focus will not matter since the intervention can be designed on this metalevel.

The conductor is going to attempt to help the family establish a goal, or goals, for the therapy that can aid in focusing tasks by relating one goal to one problem.* Usually the conductor asks the family (not an individual) a question of this type: "What do you want to accomplish in your work here with us?" Again, the conductor is likely to emphasize that different opinions about this are inevitable, but he will try to help the family narrow the focus to one goal. In helping the family focus, the conductor will attempt to assist it in clarifying its responses and in being as specific and behavioral as possible in its description of the goal. He will not push this attempt if the family shows an inability to focus, nor will he abandon his noncritical attitude.

Focusing is very important because as long as the family's goals are either too global or too distant in the future, there is no effective way for either the

---

*It must be remembered that families are generally very Aristotelian. Therefore, the conductor deals with sequences while with the family "as if" simple cause-effect rules were in operation. Families are not interested in the refinement of circular thinking no matter how epistemologically correct.

family or the team to know the usefulness of therapy. Therefore, as part of the focusing process, the conductor will ask the family about what will convince it that "significant progress is being made toward the goal?" Or, "What, at minimum, will need to happen for you to be sure the problem is on the way to solution?"

The interactional interviewing technique can also be useful when trying to establish signs of progress or goals. For instance, the conductor can ask this type of question of each person: "Mrs. H., how do you think Mr. H. will be convinced that the problem is on the way to solution?" He can then ask Mr. H. the same thing about Mrs. H. The answers to this type of question will provide the team with some information about how family members perceive each other. This type of information is an important part of the data that the team needs for reframing.

The conductor is usually rather active in helping the family define this "sign" of progress in concrete terms. For example, the family may want the thumbsucking to stop. This seems a reasonable enough goal. However, the success can never be known with certainty. Therefore, the signs of progress are necessary for both the family and the team to know if their efforts are paying off. It is easier to measure when something starts than to be sure that something has stopped because—even after a long interval—it might start again. Families will often pick a period of time as a sign that its problem is on the way to solution, that is, so many days without thumbsucking.

Client's goals can roughly be plotted along a continuum: vague to specific. The conductor will help to clarify the type of goal so that the team can phrase the goal as the start of something even if the family cannot. However, it is not always possible to find a way to help extremely vague or confused families become more specific. It is with very vague or highly confused families that the conductor will attempt to define more definite signs of progress that can be useful even if the goal remains undefined.

When the family's complaints are quite vague, its goals are more than likely to be as vague, and any signs of progress it can identify will likely be vague. At times the conductor must simply accept this vagueness as part of the family's effort to cooperate. The conductor might well renew this goal-establishing effort in later sessions because of the need for the family to know the usefulness of therapy. Of course, this vagueness is as useful to the team as any other type of information because it informs the team about how best to be isomorphic with the family's patterns.

Signs can often indicate the family's movement outside its (inferred) frame on its way toward meeting the goal of eliminating the complaint pattern. Also, the achievement of the signs (or subgoals) helps to indicate to the team that it is time to increase the interval between sessions because the frame is broken and spontaneous changes may follow as the reorganization of the system begins—a process that takes time. That is, signs are often some newly acceptable behavior that indicate that a new set of rules or definitions are starting to operate.

The conductor's noncritical stance is related to Selvini-Palazzoli's concept of "positive connotation," which involves attributing "constructive intentions to the kind of interpersonal behavior that is commonly described as destructive or injurious" (55, p. 228). However, the noncritical stance is applied to the entire situation the family describes and to its world view; it is not limited to the "problem situation." This accepting attitude helps to generate the kind of suprasystemic cooperating necessary for successful therapy. The conductor first accepts the family's patterns and the specific frames that it uses to define what it is that is going on. Only then will the family allow the team to cooperate with it in promoting change: a principle learned from Erickson.

During both the prelude and the data-collecting sections of the session, the team is doing much more than just watching another therapist work with a family. Once the team broke through the looking glass, it became more involved in the therapy than just helping the therapist when he needed it. As the team came to realize that it was a full participator in the therapy session and as it came to realize that it was part of the same suprasystem that included the family system and the therapist in the room with the family, the team realized that its roles and tasks needed to be defined so that the family could have the benefit of its collective experience.

One of the primary tasks the team defined for itself while behind the mirror is to describe the family system in such a way that developing isomorphic interventions is facilitated and that developing team–family cooperating is promoted. Since these concepts are concurrent and since they define the family interaction from different angles, a descriptive tool that includes both types of data in a way that is useful to the team is to be preferred.

Throughout the session the team is observing the patterns that the family is showing in response to the actions–reactions of the conductor. Furthermore, the team is listening for any patterns that the family members describe as occurring on a regular basis. In particular, of course, the team is interested in the patterns that are described by the family that occur around the area of the complaint. The team is interested in behavioral sequences into which these patterns fall and in the frames–meanings–beliefs that the family members attribute to the behaviors that are part of the sequence. (The interactional interviewing technique, described above, is useful to the team's effort to gather these types of data because it can elicit information about the sequence and about the frames.)

However, due to a lack of words in the English language, these patterns must be described sequentially, even though the behaviors might happen simultaneously, and various members of the family might describe the sequence as occurring in a different order. Of course, the conductor and the family, as part of a social discussion, necessarily talk about the patterns "as if" the pattern was governed by simple "cause-effect," and as if the pattern happened in a simple sequence. This type of description is sufficient as long as the team is careful to remember that the patterns are circular and multicausal.

A mapping technique has been developed to facilitate describing these patterns, including both sequence and frames, at least in a sketchy manner, that is useful in describing the patterns and in developing interventions. The classic "nag–withdraw" pattern will be used to illustrate the use of the technique. For instance, if the husband is asking his wife to tell him that she loves him and she does not and the couple describes these behaviors as repeating, then the sort of map shown in Figure 3.1 can be made.

It must be remembered that this punctuation is arbitrary, and the map could have started with "/. Wife is silent," which is the husband's punctuation. That is, when the husband describes this sequence he will explain that he asks his wife questions about her love "because she is silent and does not tell him on her own." When the wife describes this sequence, she will explain that she does not answer his repeated questions because "all he ever does is nag me." In short, he describes the sequence as "I nag because she withdraws," while she describes the sequence as "I withdraw because he nags." The couple might offer further explanations. He might say that he has to ask her repeatedly if she loves him because he feels insecure when she has not told him for some time. She, on the other hand, might say that she does not respond to his frequent questions because she becomes angry since his questions indicate to her that he does not trust her. Besides that, she might say, "Actions speak louder than words," and she does *show* him that she loves him. Some of this information can be added to the map to help the team describe the context (or frames) in which this sequence occurs (Figure 3.2).

Once the "frames" or "attributed meanings" or "the names of the context" column is added to the map of the behavioral sequence, the team can add a third column to the map that will provide it with some indication of possible ways to reframe the situation, possible different meanings the same behavioral sequence might have.* These potential new meanings are positively phrased to provide the different angle. For in-

---

*Keeping track of three columns is one of the purposes of having a team behind the mirror. It is difficult for one person (a therapist without a team) to keep track of the (1) sequence, (2) frames, and (3) potential reframes. Therefore, as a training device, these three tasks are handled separately. A trainee is first asked to keep notes about what is going on and to phrase the notes only in positive terms, which provides the conductor with material to use for reframing. Keeping track of the described behavioral sequence is the next task a trainee is assigned. In general, the sequence and the family's frames are dealt with by the conductor explicitly, and, therefore, this information is on

BEHAVIOR SEQUENCE

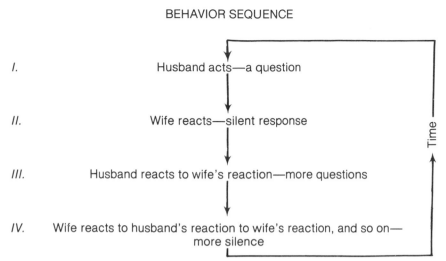

Figure 3.1.

stance, the wife's silence could be described as protecting her husband from being overwhelmed should she really express the depth of her feelings. Or, his questions could be described as protective of his wife from having doubts about his feelings while he is so frequently on the road. (These meanings are only suggestive. The reframing that the team does depends on the context, and it is not usually transferable from family to family.) The team might also include on the section of the map the individual's preferred representational system (In this particular situation). From this description, it can be inferred that the husband prefers the auditory system—he wants to *hear* the words from her—whereas the wife prefers the visual system—she wants to be *shown* (Figure 3.3).

This way of mapping an interactional sequence can be very helpful to a therapist or a team in designing interventions or reframing messages. The elements on the map (*I*, *II*, etc.) represent the concrete facts of the situation. The arrows have a double purpose: (*1*) *they stand for "leads to" and (2)* they stand for the "context" of the behavioral sequence. The "frame column" gives the names of the context that the family gives or that the team is able to infer from the family's description. The "potential meanings" column gives the team alternate names of the context that can

the recording or videotape. Since the first session's intervention tends to be broad and general, the reframing material is of primary importance. The other two columns of the map can be picked up from the tape. It is, of course, the goal of training to develop brief family therapists who can do effective work when working without a team. This mapping technique can readily be transferred to note taking when working without a team once the therapist has had enough experience.

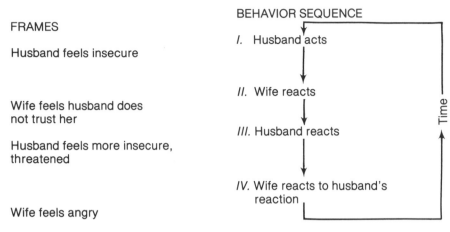

Figure 3.2.

be used for reframing purposes. When designing a reframing message, it is the arrows that are subject to transforming. Isomorphism is maintained because the elements (*I, II,* etc.) remain the same, but the meanings the team might attribute provide the therapeutic message with a "different angle," and thus the family might receive the bonus—news of a difference that can lead to change.

Furthermore, this way of mapping also describes the sequence itself. If the family's manner of cooperating is shown to include task perform-

Figure 3.3.

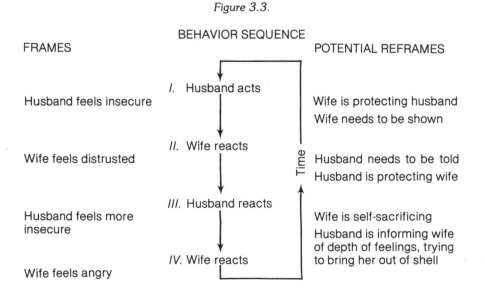

ance, then this map also provides the data about the sequence that the team can use to design tasks. (Guidelines for developing tasks will be described in Chapter 4.)

This mapping technique is not limited to couples in therapy; it can be used with larger families. For instance, the family might describe the following sequence: (*I*) the child misbehaves, then (*II*) the father yells at the child, then (*III*) the child cries while the mother intervenes, then (*IV*) mother and father argue while the child leaves the scene, then (*V*) the father resumes his disciplining of the child, and (*VI*) mother withdraws to her room. After some period of time, this sequence repeats (Figure 3.4).

The family might offer a large range of meanings for this sequence. For instance, father might yell at the child because he thinks the child needs to be taught the correct way of doing things. He might also think that mother is not strict enough about the child's behavior. Mother might not have disciplined that particular behavior because she did not think it "worth it," and she intervened because she thought father was being too strict. Therefore, mother and father argued about this disagreement, and the child cried because either (*1*) father was too harsh or (*2*) because the parents argued. Father, who thought mother was being too soft, resumes his disciplining while mother is angry with father and moves away from him.

Figure 3.4.

BEHAVIOR SEQUENCE

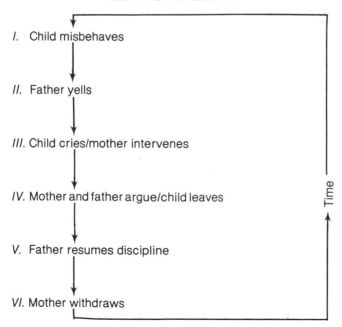

Among various alternative meanings the team might ascribe, the following might fit and be useful. Father, by disciplining the child and thus appearing as a "bad guy," might be protecting the mother's being the "good guy" and thus protecting the mother–child relationship. Mother, by intervening, might be protecting the father–child relationship by trying to help father appear less the bad guy. Furthermore, the argument between the parents might protect the child from feeling the wrath of father's anger. And, the child's misbehavior might protect the parents' marriage by pulling them together, and this might be the child's intuitive response to his perception of too great a distance between his parents. Father's returning to the discipline after the argument might be protecting mother from having to act the bad guy and, therefore, might be seen as indicating a self-sacrifice on his part since he is willing to appear the bad guy. Mother's withdrawal might be seen as protecting father's right to have a direct, open relationship with his child rather than a relationship mediated through the mother, something that happens in many families (Figure 3.5).

Figure 3.5.

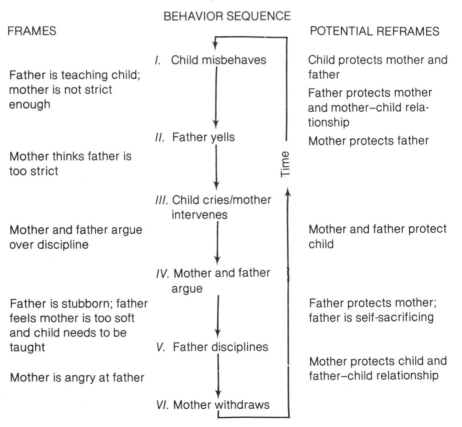

BEHAVIOR SEQUENCE

FRAMES

POTENTIAL REFRAMES

I. Child misbehaves

Father is teaching child; mother is not strict enough

Child protects mother and father

Father protects mother and mother–child relationship

II. Father yells

Mother protects father

Mother thinks father is too strict

Time

III. Child cries/mother intervenes

Mother and father argue over discipline

Mother and father protect child

IV. Mother and father argue

Father is stubborn; father feels mother is too soft and child needs to be taught

Father protects mother; father is self-sacrificing

V. Father disciplines

Mother is angry at father

Mother protects child and father–child relationship

VI. Mother withdraws

This type of mapping procedure might only be started rather sketchily in the first session, with more and more information added as the conductor is able to elicit it from the family. Regardless of the detail in the first session, this mapping technique can help the team to develop ways of being isomorphic in its interventions and can help the team infer something about the family's probable manner of cooperating. In part, this later information comes from the interview itself because the interaction between the conductor and the family indicates (enough for the team to have a good hunch about) the family's manner of cooperating. If the family shows a manner of cooperating that allows the conductor to get a lot of details, then the team can infer that tasks might be useful. If the family shows a relatively vague way of cooperating that leaves the map with few details, then the team can assume that tasks might not be useful.

This mapping technique helps to give some order to the data that give the team some understanding of the patterns, even though the details may need to be clarified or corrected as the therapy continues. Nonetheless, this approximation maintains the circular emphasis that can be useful to the team's intervention designing. This procedures has distinct advantages because the map has both "the concrete facts" that the family describes and "the context." Furthermore, this mapping procedure begins to define the different angle that the team needs to use to promote change.

THE CONSULTING BREAK:
INTERVENTION DESIGNING

The signs, the goals, and the information on the maps provide the team with the data it needs to design an intervention, which in the BFTC format has two parts: (1) the compliment and (2) the clue. As much as possible the team needs to phrase the intervention using the family's favorite phrases and predicates while keeping in mind that the intervention has to be based on a description made from a different angle. This phrasing makes it easier for the team to develop and present an intervention that is isomorphic, which makes it easier for the family to accept since it acknowledges its realities. The family seems to feel that it has been heard when the team uses its language in this manner.

The Compliment

Once the team has described the family's pattern(s) in terms of both sequence and meanings, then it can develop an intervention that builds the first steps of a "yes set" (27, 28). That is, some positive statements with which the family can agree are used to facilitate its acceptance of the clues (suggestions or tasks) that follow the compliment. This yes set is initiated by getting the family's attention focused on the conductor as he returns to the room while they wait for whatever remarks he is going to make. Then, in the first part of his statement he recognizes and acknowledges the family's current experiences (both in the therapy room and outside of it while dealing with its situation), which he is going to associate with the clue about how to start solving the family's puzzle. The yes set primarily is designed to increase the likelihood that the family will find a way to cooperate with the therapeutic suggestion or task. This likelihood is increased if the team's intervention has been designed to be isomorphic.

When the conductor returns to the room after the consulting break, the family is probably expecting a profound series of insights and interpretations about its psychological makeup. (As one client remarked: "Well, when do I hear the bad stuff?") The family might even be prepared to fight off these kinds of "negative statements" (like an opponent). Instead, the team develops complimentary statements based on the reframing section of the map and details of the family's description. Usually the first session compliment is rather general, and the compliments get more specific as the sessions continue.

For instance, if a family had provided the team with enough detail to fill in the previous map seen in Figure 3.5, then the team's compliment could be something like this:

> First of all, we are impressed with all the fine details you've given us about your situation. Most families we've met are nowhere near as observant of these details. Your descriptions have been very helpful to us. It's clear to us that you are both loving and dedicated parents who've been resourceful in trying to find ways to solve the problem. Another unusual thing struck us: You each seem to care a lot about how the other parent treats the boy. Many parents would be only interested in the boy's difficulties.

This compliment includes the second step in building a yes set, which is fixing the family's attention on their current experiences. The third step is to relate indirectly the family's current experiences with the clue.

The Clue

This part of the intervention, the clue, should utilize the behavioral sequence section of the map, while still being as isomorphic as possible. The clearer the behavioral sequence has been described, the easier it is for the team to develop a task.

For instance, with the same family, the conductor could continue with the following:

> Between now and next time we meet, the team would like you each to observe what happens when you are alone with Jimmie and he misbehaves like this. And we would like to know some other details: When during the

week—which days and what time—does Jim most frequently misbehave while both of you are there.

Most clues, like this one, are associated with something to be expected reasonably in the immediate future, that is, the child's continuing misbehavior. Often these "contingent suggestions can be tied together into associational networks that create a system of mutual support and momentum for initiating and carrying out a therapeutic pattern of responses" (27, p. 33). That is, if the family has accepted the compliment, there is a likelihood that it will find the associated task or suggestion to be within its manner of cooperating. Case examples throughout will illustrate the use of this yes set or combination of a compliment and a clue as the form of the intervention. This intervention set allows the team to operationalize the concurrent concepts of isomorphism and cooperating.

Once the intervention is designed, the conductor will rehearse reading it or presenting it if it is not written down. After about 10 minutes, the conductor will return to the therapy room.

MESSAGE GIVING

While the conductor is delivering the intervention, the team is watching how each of the family members reacts to the messages. Frequently, the family members will show their acceptance by nodding to some of the points the conductor mentions (hence the label "yes set"). If the message is really built on an isomorphic description, the family will sometimes build upon the ideas with further examples that indicate the team has understood the patterns.

However, if the family does not show its acceptance of the compliment, the conductor can build additional points based on the data on the map. The team may phone in further points or it may suggest that the conductor *not* deliver the planned clue. If the family does not accept the compliment, then it is not likely to find a way to cooperate with the clue. If the family fails to show signs of accepting the compliment, this is information that means that the team's description probably was not isomorphic enough.

Once the conductor is relatively sure that the family has accepted the compliment, he continues with the delivery of the clue. After that, he gives the family a little time to clarify the suggestions and to react to the whole message. However, other discussion is held to a minimum so that the associational network can develop the momentum for the family to carry out a therapeutic response. Other topics and new information can interfere with this process, so the conductor moves quickly to end the session.

STUDY EFFORTS

After the family has left, the team meets to access the family's immediate responses to the message and then to predict the type of responses to the task that the family is likely to report in the next session.

First, the team will note its observations of the family's responses to the compliment and clue. From this, the team will make some predictions. If the family showed its acceptance, the team will predict that the family will return for the next session. Then the team will make predictions about the type of response the family will report to the clue: Will it perform the task in a straightforward manner, or will it modify it, or will it do the opposite of it, or will it not do the task, or will the response report be too vague for the team to know (see Chapter 4). If the team has found the family's manner of cooperating and the compliment and clue were isomorphic enough, then the team's ability to predict will be closer to the mark.

Second, the team will make predictions about the likelihood that the family will either report changes in the complaint pattern or that it will show the team some changes in the next session. All of these predictions are kept as part of the team's record.

The team often gets the best results when it is experimenting without any specific result in mind as a goal for a particular intervention. The signs and goals give the team a direction in which to move but not information on how to get there. The "how to get there" comes more from the responses to the messages that the family will report in the following session. Particularly with the initial clue, the team is *not* looking for a particular result, but rather it is looking for which one of the set of probable results will occur. The main results of the first session's messages is the information the family's response report will provide.

Chapter 4 will deal specifically with the response report patterns and the construction of tasks. Chapter 4 and the subsequent chapters will deal with more complex and vague family patterns than were dealt with in this chapter on the procedures in the first session. Since the same type of information is needed and the message-constructing method is the same, the format of the later sessions remains unchanged. The principal data to be collected center around the family's response report to the task that gives the team a progressively more useful description of the family's unique manner of cooperating. This information will allow more precision in task designing.

CHAPTER 4

More Procedures

INTERCONNECTIONS

Chapter 3 described the procedures used in the first session. In the later sessions the format remains the same, and many of the same procedures are used. Once a family returns for a second session, the team will have more information about the manner of cooperating that the family shows, and thus the team will be better able to cooperate with the family's efforts to change. Each subsequent intervention is built upon the reported results of the previous message, and therefore the team's description will map more and more closely onto the family's patterns.

Since we cannot follow the family with a candid camera crew throughout the interval between sessions, we cannot detail the mechanism of the family's reaction to the intervention. Even with the candid camera technique, we still might not have any assurance that we are dealing with a simple "cause-effect" relationship between intervention and change, an idea that too easily becomes lineal, which is not useful in an ecosystemic situation. In the therapy situation, we can only control—to the best of our ability—the therapeutic interventions.

Perhaps we need not be as concerned about cause and effect as it may at first appear. As Capra has suggested, "the structures and phenomena we observe in nature are nothing but creatures of our measuring and categorizing mind" (13, p. 266). Subatomic physicists can only observe the results of their experiments in high speed collisions by studying the photographs of what has already happened. The physicists have developed S-matrix theory diagrams that do not picture the detailed mechanisms of a reaction but merely specify the initial and final particles. Thus, the S matrix "is a collection of probabilities for all possible reactions involving hadrons" (13, p. 266).

> The important new concept in S-matrix theory is the shift of emphasis from objects to events; its basic concern is not with particles, but with their reactions. Such a shift from objects to events is required by both quantum theory and relativity theory. On the one hand, quantum theory has made it clear that a subatomic particle can only be understood as a manifestation of the

interaction between various processes of measurement. It is not an isolated object, but rather an occurrence, or event, which interconnects with other events in a particular way. . . . . The interconnections in such a network cannot be determined with certainty, but are associated with probabilities. Each reaction occurs with some probability. (13, pp. 252, 254)

Although subatomic physics can only loosely be applied as a metaphor to the therapy situation, nonetheless the shift from objects to events and to multicasual processes is similar. We are not studying people, or families, or therapy as objects. Rather, we are studying the interactions between the subsystems of an ecosystem. We are looking for events and processes that indicate there are interconnections between the series of events in the first session and the series of events in the second session: the initial state (during the first session) of the family system, then an intervention, then a period of time, followed by a new state that the family will show the team in the second session. Each therapy session can be considered an independent "experiment" with the following session as a measurement of the new state achieved since the prior session. We can record the indicated interconnections without considering the intervention as "causitive" in the traditional sense.

Of course, the therapist (as scientist/craftsman) needs to view the intervention and change as interconnective, otherwise therapy would be meaningless chaos and chance. This assumption can be mitigated by the knowledge that this is not a simple cause–effect relationship, but rather it is a part of a multicausal chain. This multicausal chain is too complex to be studied in a linear fashion. The multicausal chain could be described in this fashion: (1) the family describes its situation to the therapy team; (2) the team makes a map describing that description; based on that description (of the family's description), (3) the team designs an intervention (isomorphically and in line with the expected manner of cooperating); (4) the family receives the intervention; (5) during the interval between sessions, the family reacts to the intervention and to its daily life situations; (6) the family returns to the therapy where it describes its reaction to the intervention and to its life situation; and (7) the team describes the family's description, and so forth. Thus we can follow the patterns of the family and therapy-team subsystems and the interactions of the suprasystem as a process or series of observed events that keeps in mind the relationship of the observer to the observed. In this way, the second session (6, above) is similar to the photographs of the events that physicists study (Figure 4.1). Neither the physicist nor the brief family therapist can know the details of the complex mechanisms that occurred between event 1 and event 2. The S matrix can only provide the physicist with a probablity for each of the possible outcomes. Brief family therapists can also know that each outcome occurs with some probability (Figure 4.2).

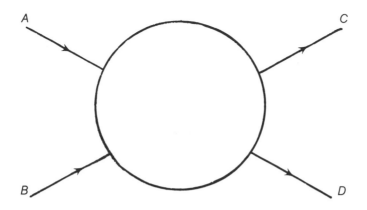

Figure 4.1. S-matrix diagram (after Capra). "Hadron processes . . . are represented symbolically by diagrams like the one above which pictures one of the simplest and most general particle reactions: A and B undergo a collision and emerge as two different particles, C and D. These diagrams . . . do not picture the detailed mechanism of the reaction, but merely specify the initial and final particles" (13, pp. 250-251).

TASKS

Since a large number of family therapy models and brief therapy models includes the use of tasks, directives, or assignments as part of their method of intervening, it seems rather curious that very little material is available to guide therapists in the construction of specific interventions that may include tasks for the family to perform between therapy sessions.

Various authors inlcuding Haley (38), Minuchin (49), Watzlawick *et al.* (64), and de Shazer (20, 21, 24) discuss the value and use of tasks in therapy. It seems that "the practice of giving instructions to patients is a form of behavior at least as ancient as the concept of healing itself" (1, p. 96). Tasks are often "a form of strategic intervention that serves several purposes. In general, the assignment of a task is used *to promote change,* that is to activate new transactional patterns" (1, p. 99).

Haley gives some additional purposes:

> Giving directives, or tasks, to individuals and families has several purposes. First, the main goal of therapy is to get people to behave differently and so to have different subjective experiences. Directives are a way of making those changes happen. Second, directives are used to intensify the relationship with the therapist. . . . Third, directives are used to gather information. (38, p. 49)

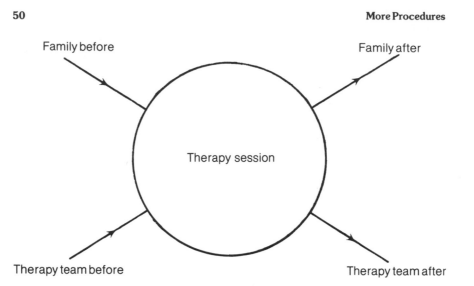

Figure 4.2. S-matrix diagram. The therapy session is represented symbolically by the above diagram. The family system and the therapy team undergo a collision, with the purpose of changing the family. This diagram does not picture the detailed mechanism of the therapy session but merely specifies the initial and final states of both the team and the family.

The clinical experience is that some people will perform tasks, and others will not. Some information is available from the field of pharmacology that indicates, on the average, people only take about half the dosages prescribed for them, and in some instances people fail to take as much as 90% of prescribed medications (11). Although similar research does not seem to have been done in the family therapy field, there is no reason to assume that psychotherapy research would produce significantly dissimilar results for the field as a whole.

For most family therapists, the attitude toward task completion seems to be that

> sometimes a family accepts a task and finds that the alternative behaviors elicited by it are preferable to the old ones—that the family can function better in the expanded range. At other times family members modify the task, contradict it, or avoid it. (49, p. 152)

When the family does not perform the task, most models suggest that the family is showing resistance to change. This notion can be seen as a failure on the therapist's part to punctuate the situation in such a way that "noncompliance" can be seen as a product of the interactional situation—the suprasystem. Whatever the family's response to the tasks, its report provides therapists with new information that clarifies the situation.

Some authors have made suggestions for increasing the likelihood that a family will accept the task and then perform it. Along with the MRI group (64), de Shazer has suggested phrasing tasks in the family's "language" so that the task fits better into the family's world view (19). This will make it easier for the family to accept the directive.

The brief family therapy model suggests that the family's response to a task is a product of the interaction and communication between the two subsystems, and its response is a message about the relationship between the two subsystems. Furthermore, the family's reported response is a message to the team about how it is showing its unique manner of cooperating. Therefore, any response the family reports can be placed into one of five categories (straightforward, modified, opposite, vague, or nil) and is part of the family's pattern and part of the suprasystem's pattern. From this point of view, all tasks are successful because they provide the therapist with more information about the differences between his maps and the family's way of cooperating that it is showing him.

To what degree did the family or the individual family members perform the task? Does the family report any changes? Does the team observe any changes? What do the changes look like? Are the changes observed or reported by the family in line with the team's predictions? All of these questions and the answers are necessary information for the team to have before the next intervention is designed. Thus, gathering this information is the primary concern of the conductor during the "data-collecting" section of the session. The families' reported responses—(1) straightforward, (2) modified, (3) opposite, (4) vague, or (5) nil—indicate to the therapist which type of response the therapist needs to make so that he can cooperate with a particular family.

Response Report-Intervention Patterns

1. If the family were given a direct task as part of the clue and the family reports having performed the task in a straightforward manner as given by the team, then the model suggests that the next therapeutic intervention include another direct task. The family has shown that its manner of cooperating includes the performance of direct tasks, and, therefore, the team can continue cooperating by using another direct task to help promote change.

For instance, the Shack family was given the task to observe and record the frequency of arguments, fights, or hassles between their two boys (six and eight years old). In the second session, the family's report included dates, times, and places of the fights for each day during the two-week interval. The parents noted that the frequency and duration of the hassles diminished as the interval came to a close. Their reports also indicated that mother intervened more frequently than father, even though father was at home at the time.

Since the family reported a straightforward response to the first task, the team designed another straightforward task: Mother and father were asked to alternate days on which they each were to be solely in charge of handling the boys' hassles and fights. The other parent was to observe and to remain as detached as possible. The team predicted that the Shack family would perform this task. And the third session report indicated that the Shack family did follow through in a straightforward manner, and that the frequency and duration of the hassles both diminished regardless of which parent intervened.

2. If the family reports modifying a direct task, then the model suggests that the team continue cooperating by giving the family a task that can be easily modified. Sometimes the team can spell out these options to the family, or the team can give the family an indirect task within the clue (such as by telling a story that has a pattern that is isomorphic with the family's patterns). The family may report a response that indicates that it modified an indirect task into a direct task. That is, its report will be presented to the team in such a way that the family shows it was following a directive.

For instance, Mr. Rose was given the task to observe what happened between his wife and his son when she caught the boy in one of his frequent lies. Mrs. Rose was given the reverse of the task: She was to observe what happened when Mr. Rose caught the boy. They were asked to do this each evening between supper time and the boy's bedtime. In the second session, they reported doing the task in a much more random fashion.

Since the family reported a modification of a direct task, the team designed an intervention that would easily allow the family to cooperate by again modifying the task. The parents were told a story about how another family with a little liar achieved a miracle cure. Each time the mother observed father dealing with the boy about a lie, she would give the child a penny, and the father did the same when he observed mother and son dealing together about lies. These parents were careful to do this irregularly and not to say a word when giving their child a penny. For some reason, the lies stopped. After this story, Mr. and Mrs. Rose were told to keep track of how often their son lied during the next two weeks. The team predicted that Mr. and Mrs. Rose would adopt some version of the "penny trick."

When the family returned for the next session, they reported that they "had followed the team's advice" and gave the boy a penny whenever they caught him dealing with the other parent about a lie. At first the boy seemed confused, and then they were horrified when the lies increased for a day, but they stuck with the advice. Three days after the lies reached their peak, they suddenly stopped. They had not caught the boy in a lie for 10 days in a row.

Comment. This sort of intervention or gimmick is often erroneously labeled a "paradoxical intervention." However, it is not paradoxical. The intervention can be mapped in a straightforward manner upon the family's pattern and its reported response to the previous task. The family's patterns are not described as paradoxical, and, therefore, the intervention cannot be labeled a paradoxical intervention because there is no paradox for the intervention to counter.

As Dell points out (17), just because the result was not what should be expected when using Aristotelian premises, it does not make the intervention paradoxical.

> When a problem remains unchanged in the face of an attempted solution,
> Westerners do not conclude that their premises are incorrect. Instead, they
> decide that the problem is serious and persistent. This interpretation is con-
> sidered to be "common sense." Easterners, however, would conclude that
> the *solution* was inappropriate. For them, the reality of the situation lies in
> the interaction between the "problem" and the attempted solution. This is
> also the view of the interactional therapist. "Common sense," apparently,
> is relative to one's "culture." (17, p. 40)

The therapist using this type of intervention expects the outcome: an end to the boy's lies and an end to the parent's interaction with him around lies. Therefore, to the therapist this intervention does not sound "absurd" or paradoxical, although it may seem so to the family (who can be seen to use Aristotelian premises).

3. If the family reports doing the opposite of a direct task, then the model suggests that the team can best continue cooperating with the family's way of cooperating by giving the family a task that includes the potential for "opposite" responses.

For instance, Mrs. Ribbon spent the whole first session detailing her complaints about her husband and her relationship with him. Recently the abusive nature of the situation had worsened, but Mrs. Ribbon rejected the idea of separating. The team gave her the task to "think about, and to write down, what you do *not* want to see change about your husband and your relationship with him." Although she appeared puzzled, she agreed to do the task.

When she returned for the second session, she reported that she was only able to think about what was *wrong,* and, therefore, she had moved out. At this point she felt elated and saw things through rose-colored glasses, which she did not allow to interfere with thinking about the practical steps she needed to take.

Since she had reported an "opposite response" to the first task, the team gave her a task based on this information. The team suggested that when most people split up a marriage, they soon get very depressed and start to think about getting back together. Therefore, the team asked Mrs. Ribbon to watch for signs that she was getting depressed and to keep notes about this.

When she returned for the third session, she reported nothing but positives, and, therefore, she had kept track of the good things that had happened. She did not see any signs of a developing depression and thought that the team was wrong in its assessment of her situation.

4. If the family's report on its response to a direct task is vague and/or confused, then the team can best continue cooperating with the pattern the family has shown by designing and giving a vague task. Frequently this vagueness is shown to the team during the first session's discussion of goals. Nonetheless, the team usually gives a direct task so that the second session report can clarify this situation. In many situations, vagueness will follow vagueness until the family demands clarity. Then the team needs to respond with clarity.

For instance, Mr. and Mrs. Glass were unable to specify a goal for therapy beyond "better communication." They would know that this had happened when they both "felt better." At no time during the first session were they able to describe any behavior changes that would indicate either better communication or better feelings. In fact, questions about behavioral changes led to further descriptions of vague feelings of discomfort. The team asked Mr. and Mrs. Glass to observe what was going on when they experienced these feelings of discomfort or when they experienced a block in communication.

During the second session, Mr. and Mrs. Glass reported on how they experienced their reactions to the communication block and how thinking about the bad feelings had made them aware of "just how bad they felt." Neither of them was able to describe what was going on between them that prompted these feelings. The team asked Mr. and Mrs. Glass to "notice when they first started to get these feelings of discomfort, and then to *do* something different." Then the team asked them to "report on how doing something different made them feel better."

During the third session, Mr. and Mrs. Glass both reported feeling better. Mrs. Glass attributed this to the therapy team, which suggested to her that she could choose between "good or bad feelings." After congratulating them on this discovery, the team suggested that the bad feelings are likely to return or to once again be predominant in their experience. Furthermore, the team suggested that this relapse "would give you further experience in choosing good over bad feelings."

The couple reported in the next session that both of them felt better than they had in recent years. Therapy terminated with this session.

Comment. At no point during the therapy were any behavioral goals or signs of progress established. In this type of situation it is always difficult for the team to *know* that therapy was successful, except through clients' reports. However, the team can develop isomorphic interventions or messages that are as vague as the family's information. Keeping in mind that these messages are presented to the family "from a different angle," the family can still receive the desired bonus of change. Since the family patterns and the interventions are vague, naturally the outcome will be vague.

5. If the family reports not doing a direct task (for whatever reason), this may mean either (a) that not doing tasks is part of the family's manner of cooperating, which it is showing the team or (b) that the team's map of the family's pattern of cooperating as shown in the first session was not close enough to be isomorphic. In either case, the team needs to redefine its understanding of the family patterns. Then a direct task can be given as "an experiment" to test the team's new description. If the family subsequently reports performing the experiment, then the team's new description probably was more isomorphic. However, if the family reports *not* performing the experiment, then this probably shows the team that performing tasks is not part of the family's manner of cooperating. In either case, the response report provides the team with more information about how to be isomorphic and how best to continue cooperating. Even without direct tasks, change can be promoted through messages that are isomorphic enough to give the family the desired bonus. Of course, the team can continue cooperating by not giving tasks, or they can use stories (see 2, above). The family need not *do* anything to cooperate since it is not being directly asked to *do* anything.

(This method can be used effectively with reluctant families or even with involuntary clients.)

For instance, Mr. and Mrs. King and their daughter Janet (aged 14) complained about what happens when Janet did not get her way. Aside from frequent tantrums, Janet would sometimes run out of the house and stay out too late. The family was asked to keep track of when, where, and who was involved in these hassles during the interval between sessions.

During the second session no member of the King family was able to report on these details. Shortly after the first session, Janet had a "big tantrum," and this disturbed everyone. Although there were other tantrums during the week, nobody could remember when they happen or who was involved. Mr. and Mrs. King continued to detail their complaints about Janet's behavior. As the session continued, it became clear to the team that the King family was showing that they considered the problem to "reside in Janet" and that Mr. and Mrs. King were not going to perform any tasks since that would imply that they agreed that *they* needed to change. As far as Mr. and Mrs. King were concerned, Janet had the problem and she needed to change. Equally, Janet showed the team that she was not going to change. The team apologized for having given them the wrong homework in the previous session. And the team suggested that they were glad the King family had not gone ahead with the tasks since that probably would have made things worse. The team complimented them on their descriptions of the complicated situation in which they found themselves and suggested that it—the team—had misunderstood the serious nature of Janet's difficulties. The session ended with these statements.

The complaints about Janet's misbehavior continued into the third session. The family reported no change. The team suggested to Mr. and Mrs. King that, although Janet was clearly having big problems, an experiment on their part might help the team clarify the true nature of the problem. Therefore, the team asked Mr. and Mrs. King to do something different—it did not matter what—next time Janet had a temper tantrum. Janet's response would help the team determine just "what kind of problem" Janet did have. (The team did not expect Mr. and Mrs. King to perform the experiment. This was designed just to test the team's description of the King family's manner of cooperating.)

During the following session, Mr. and Mrs. King reported having been unable to think of anything different to do, and, therefore, they did not do the experiment. (This clarified for the team the manner of cooperating that the King family was showing.) The team designed an intervention that would not call for any of the King family to perform a task. In this message, the team stated that Janet's problems were (a) an immature attempt to keep her parents intimately involved with her childish misbehavior and (b) likely to continue until it was proved to her that her parents would still be intensely involved with her when the problems stopped. Both of these points were elaborated upon in great length, and no task was given.

During the three-week interval between sessions, Janet's tantrums diminished in frequency and intensity. This did not seem to change the number of the parents' complaints. After another two weeks, the number of complaints had also dropped as the frequency of tantrums declined.

Comment. This fifth category of patterns of response can be the most difficult for the team to respond to with isomorphic messages. At first it is usually unclear if the "nonperformance" is a message to the team that they did not have a good description of the family's probable manner of cooperating or if the nonperformance is what the family is showing about its manner of cooperating. An experimental task is often an effective way of clarifying the meaning of the message.

The fifth category is one that can prompt paradoxical interventions. The

King family's patterns can be described as including the message: "Help us change/we will not do anything to help you help us change." This statement, inferred by the team, is clearly self-reflexive. The second part—inferred from nonperformance of the tasks—is described as "meta" to the first part of the statement: It comments about itself on a different level. The intervention can then be described as counterparadoxical since the team's message just "explains" the problematic behavior and then suggests that nothing can be done until the problem is solved. The team suggests that the only way to solve the problem is for the parents to prove that they are still involved once the problem is solved. That is, the team is telling the family *not* to change until it has changed: a mirror image of the team's description of the King family's message.

However, these conceptual gymnastics are not necessary. The concepts of cooperating and isomorphism suggest a different explanation. The King family showed the team that task performance was not part of its manner of cooperating, and, therefore, the team could best cooperate by not giving tasks. The isomorphic intervention can be mapped, from a different angle, onto the family's patterns so that the family can get the bonus of change. The behavioral changes that followed show that there is some interconnection between the message and the changes.

Flow Chart or Decision Tree

These clinical vignettes illustrate the patterns of response report - intervention. As vignettes, the examples only sketch the patterns that will be explored in more detail. The patterns can be charted (as illustrated in Figure 4.3) to help the therapist decide what is the best therapeutic pattern of cooperating.

Reading the Chart. At the end of the first session, the family is given a compliment and a clue based on the team's description of the family's patterns during the first session and on the team's temporary description of the way the family will show its manner of cooperating. Based on the premise that tasks can be useful in promoting change, the first session clue is most frequently a direct task. The reported response that the family presents in the next session is information about the difference between the team's temporary description and the manner the family shows.

If the family performs the direct task in a straightforward manner and gives this report in the next session, then the team can further promote team-family cooperating by following this lead (Figure 4.3, column 1) with another direct task. (See example 1, above.) This intervention will produce *some* response (bottom of column 1), which will be reported in the next session.

The reported response in the third session is again read at the top of the chart (Figure 4.3), and the appropriate column is followed: If the response is

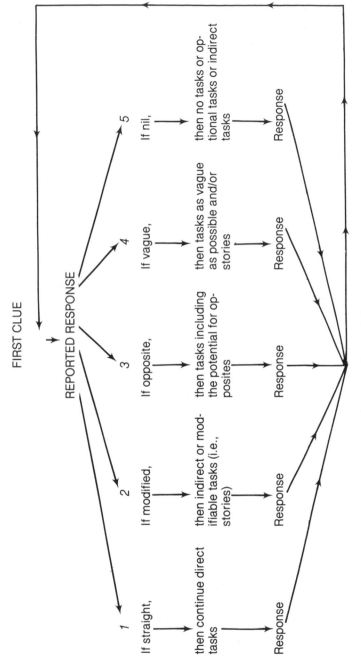

Figure 4.3.

straightforward, then the team returns to column 1; if the family modified the task, then the team switches to column 2; if the family reports doing the opposite, then the team switches to column 3; if the family report is vague or confused; then the team switches to column 4; if the family reports not doing a task, then the team switches to column 5.

If the family is given an indirect or modifiable task (for instance, a story) and its report indicates that it modified that into a direct task, then the team can switch to column 1 and give the family a direct task.

Or, if the family was given a vague task (column 4) and its returns with concrete data or demand clarity, then the team can continue cooperating by switching to column 1. This is similar to Erickson's "confusion technique" (35), which adds confusion until the subject demands clarity (see Chapter 5). That is, the team, by cooperating with the family's vagueness, has intervened in such a way that it has changed the family's manner of cooperating as shown by the switch in the family's reported response.

Of course, this flow chart or decision tree (Figure 4.3) is only a guide to assist the therapist in determining what category of task to design. How to design tasks is beyond this simple chart and will be dealt with subsequently. What is important to recognize here is that the family's response report shows the team how best to continue cooperating with the family's manner of cooperating. This is a communication about the developing patterns of the suprasystem. Tasks are not just plugged in depending on the whim of the therapist. Rather, the task is built upon the information based on the pattern of response that the family showed. Somewhat like the red light on the dashboard, the family's report tells the therapist what action he needs to take next to keep the suprasystem headed toward the desired outcome.

Designing Tasks

Various therapists seem to agree that designing effective tasks for use in family therapy is difficult because the plan should encompass not only the troublesome behavior of an individual (the traditional symptom), but it should also include the entire family interaction pattern that surrounds the troublesome behavior. Furthermore, this model suggests that the patterns of the suprasystem must be taken into account.

The Milan Group (54) described a "family ritual," a one-time-only task that seems designed to undermine dramatically the family's need for a symptom. It noted that this sort of task is uniquely tailored to a particular family system and needs to be isomorphic on various levels. These family rituals are difficult to invent, and they are not reusable with other families—no matter how similar the therapists' descriptions may be. More recently the group described a "ritual prescription" (57) that is usable with many families that includes one or more troublesome children. Except for minor details, this prescription does not vary from family to family. Importantly, the Milan group deals with the usefulness to the team of a family's noncompliance. Papp (51) described "prescribing the system," which is a "paradoxical intervention" that instructs the family to continue doing what it is already doing but to do so for the good of the family rather than because it cannot help it. Haley (38), Minuchin (49), Andolfi (1), Watzlawick et al. (64), and de Shazer (19, 20, 22, 24) all describe the use of tasks in promoting change.

Effective tasks seem to follow certain metapatterns (or patterns of patterns). Goffman (31) has studied the process of changing "serious" activities into "playful" activities. From his study of frames and how to change frames, he developed some guidelines for this transformation that can be used as a metapattern. These guidelines can be used in whole (24) or in part to help the therapist design effective tasks. The purpose of these guidelines is to help the therapist keep his designs based on the family's patterns in a modified form and in a different context.

Guidelines

1. The playful acts are so performed that their ordinary, serious functions are not realized. Efforts are made to equalize the strength of the "players."
2. There is an exaggeration of some normal acts.
3. The normal sequence serves as a pattern that is neither followed faithfully nor fully but is subject to arbitrary starting and stopping.
4. The activities called for are repetitive.
5. Any player has the power to terminate play once begun.
6. During the play the dominance order may become mixed up or reversed.
7. The play seems independent of any external needs of the participants and continues longer than would the actual interactions it is patterned after.
8. The play is social in that it involves more than one participant, and the playfulness therefore can be more easily sustained.
9. Signs are available to mark the beginning and the termination of playfulness. (adapted from 31, pp. 41-43)

Once the family's manner of cooperating has been shown to the therapist, these guidelines can be used to assist task designing. The family's pattern, the behavioral sequence as mapped, must form the basis of this type of intervention. The "concrete facts" of the pattern surrounding the complaint must be used, and these guidelines can help the therapist decide how to modify the sequence and the context in which the pattern is performed. In other words, Goffman's guidelines (31) can be used to help the therapist reframe the behavioral sequence by changing parts of the sequence. Case material will illustrate this reframing process and the use of the flow chart or decision tree.

CHANGING KEYS

It may seem a commonplace thought that small changes are easier to make than large ones. But therapists and families alike are often forced to accept small changes as the "only thing possible," sort of "second best." This is often the attitude expressed by observers of brief family therapy. The observer may see the team carefully and deliberately work toward a small change—a sign of progress—and consider his work successful when there is a small change in the frame around a family's puzzle. This aspect of brief family therapy often surprises the observers. They wonder, sometimes out loud: "How can a team of therapists consider such a minor change as significant to the family and the family's problem"?

But small changes that start the reframing process often have larger results: the solution of the puzzle when the goal is reached. Once the small change is achieved, the family is then able to perceive the complaint pattern in a different way, thus they received a bonus.

The systemic concept of wholism and Bateson's "self-healing tautology" (9) suggest that if any aspect of the system is changed, the whole organization of the system is thereby changed; each aspect of the system implies the remainder of the system. This sort of reorganization takes time, and the therapist needs to respect this time, which varies from family to family. The Milan group has adopted standard one-month intervals because of the time reorganization seems to take (56).

As an analogy, musical composition can help to make this notion about the effects of small changes clearer. Like any other human endeavor, music has rules and patterns that the composer follows either consciously or unconsciously. As we listen to music, we perceive the sequence of notes that either sounds pleasing to our ears or does not. Once we know a particular sequence of notes, any deviation will immediately let us know that something is different. Much more so for the composer since he can "know" that something is "wrong" when he is constructing the sequence. As an experiment, we can imagine that J.S. Bach might have composed the sequence shown in Figure 4.4.

These notes follow a specific sequence: F-A-B-C-A-D-C-B-A. If you were to play this sequence on a piano, you would notice that it calls for the use of only white keys. We can hear this melody as either pleasing or not pleasing.

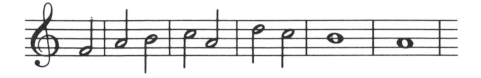

Figure 4.4.

Like any sequence of human endeavor, we perceive this music as either effective or not effective. If we perceive the music as "not quite right," then we (as experimental composors) can change it.

If we can imagine that Bach did compose this sequence in this fashion and he found it lacking, then various changes are possible. The various notes (or behaviors) in the sequence could be changed (i.e., a C could be substituted for the D) or the key could be changed (a context name), which might be the easiest and quickest approach. In fact, Bach did write this sequence, but with one small change *at the start* of the sequence, as shown in Figure 4.5.

Because of this change in key (or context) the notes follow a slightly different order: F-A-*B-flat*-C-A-D-C-*B-flat*-A. Bach's little change in the key affects the melody (behavior). That is, using B-flat instead of B made the music more effective for him. Comparing the two versions of the melody, we hear a different piece of music, which changes our whole perception of the sequence. However, it is not just a simple matter that B-flat has replaced B in the sequence that makes it different. Rather, the whole sound (context) of the melody is very different, and thus our appreciation is different. Like Bach we might find this change effective, or we might not.

If we can imagine that Bach made this same step in composing this melody, then anything he wrote after this sequence is also going to have been affected profoundly by the change of key. This small change will effect the harmony (a part of the context) and other related notes in the total composition (behavior). By adding the B-flat sign (a very small change or news of a differ-

Figure 4.5.

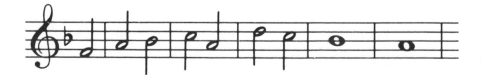

ence), Bach was able to find the simplest way of changing the musical meaning of the sequence of notes and our experience of it.

By changing the key Bach did something similar to what a therapist does when he starts the reframing process by helping a family make a small change at the "beginning" of a sequence of interaction (i.e., the complaint pattern). The whole sequence is no longer the same. Everytime the note on the middle line is to be played, it is B-flat, which is a half-tone lower than B. The outcome of this change will be perceived throughout the entire piece of music, not only in this brief melody, but in the harmony that surrounds it.

The composer had other alternatives for making a change in this sequence. Any of the individual notes in the sequence might have been changed, but adding the flat sign at the start (changing the key, or context—not just a note) was one of the easiest changes to make. In the brief family therapy arena, the process of changing keys through the isomorphic intervention is the easiest way possible. A change of key tells the musician to play differently and tells the listener to perceive the music in a different way. In therapy, changing the key starts to change the context by changing a behavior that therefore changes the entire meaning. However, this change of key is not always a simple task for the brief family therapist and probably is not a simple task for the composer either.

Wholism. Music is like any system: If you make one change, other changes will naturally follow. The changes from B to B-flat did more than just lower the tone played on the middle line of the staff by one half-step. In the musical system this change in key also "changes the relationships" among all of the notes in the composition as a whole. For instance, there are three half-steps between D and B, whereas there are four half-steps between D and B-flat. There is always this half-step difference between the notes in the two sequences: one more half-step when going down the scale toward B-flat, and one less when going up toward B-flat.

In the musical system the results of this change from B to B-flat always has the same predictable results. D is always D. At least in Bach's musical language, there is no chance that when you change B to B-flat that the next note will fall between the piano keys and be something "not quite D." A note cannot be $3\frac{1}{2}$ half-steps away from another note.

On the other hand, human interaction sequences are not that predictable. A sequence, once established, does follow certain patterns (or metapatterns) and is—within certain limits—rather predictable. The bits of behavior that seem to be able to replace each other within a sequence usually can be described as belonging to the same class of behaviors. Spanking a child, yelling at a child, or grounding a child are all bits of behavior that can be described as members of the same class: a class that might be called "disciplinary behaviors."

When brief family therapists promote change by changing the key, they help the family to add some bit of behavior from a new class at the beginning of the complaint pattern. But the changes in the sequence that will follow are not always predictable. The only sure thing is that the sequence cannot remain the same. By their very nature (perhaps) or at least by the very nature of our descriptions, interactional sequences are usually described as redundant. These sequences appear rigid in that only behaviors from the same class "spontaneously" replace each other. When a key change is introduced, the new behavior acts as if it opens up the doors for any random bit of behavior, a behavior from a different class. The key change "destroys" the sequence and introduces chance or randomness into the interaction. A new behavior might get a response 3½ half-steps away from the original, a note that is in the cracks between the piano keys. Of course, the new behavior the key change elicits is limited by the range of possible behaviors the individual brings into the situation. Although two families might start a "new sequence" with a squirt of a squirt gun, the resulting sequences may very well be different. Even though the team's maps of the families' patterns are very similar and the team decides to use a key change as part of an intervention, the results may be very different.

A CASE EXAMPLE

The key change technique can be an effective tool with couples (or larger families) when the sequence of behavior is clear and the team has discovered that the couple's manner of cooperating includes reporting responses of a straightforward nature to direct tasks. Mr. and Mrs. Harper had recently moved to the city from a rural township. One of the major reasons for this move was that Mr. Harper started to get a reputation for violence, and Mrs. Harper became embarrassed by the thought that everyone considered the violence her fault. Since Mr. Harper had lived in the area throughout his life, the sudden violence at home was believed to be Mrs. Harper's fault. Outside the home, Mr. Harper was a meak, mild-mannered man who "wouldn't hurt a fly."

Session 1

During the session Mr. Harper was apologetic while Mrs. Harper nagged him to accept the blame for once again breaking his promise to avoid violence. From his perspective, if she were the least bit predictable, then the violence would not happen. He was sorry, but he could not live with the erratic methods of running a house that his wife used: One day when he came home dinner would be on the table ready to eat; other days, the meal would be hours late. From her point of view, he was unpredictable. One day he would complain about the meal's being late, and, therefore, the next day she would have it ready when he got home. Then he would complain about the meal being ready because it did not give him a chance to relax and read the paper before eating. He apologized for putting this kind of strain on her, but he could not predict what kind of day he would have at work.

Three days before coming to therapy, the meal was late. When Mr. Harper got home from work he was angry about a pending strike and the fact that he had predicted, on the way home, that the meal would not be ready. Therefore, when he walked in the door, he had an angry look on his face. Mrs. Harper had just paid the newspaper carrier more than she thought she owed, and therefore she had an angry look on her face. They yelled and screamed at each other for a half-hour when suddenly he pushed her down and threatened to strangle her. The telephone rang and the sequence came to an end—a mild version of their usual violent episodes.

They stated their goals clearly. Both wanted the violence to stop: She wanted him to start controlling himself, and he wanted her to be more organized. She was sure that if he were to come in the front door with an angry look on his face *and* no violence followed (a sure sign of progress), then they would be on their way to a better marriage. He too wanted to be met at the door without anger when he felt anger at something "outside their marriage." They also wanted to settle the questions of "why" there was violence and of "whose fault" the violence really was.

They described their move to the city with a lot of humor, which belied the hassles they went through. They also described playing practical jokes on each other, which they both enjoyed. During the move they had several arguments that did not lead to violence, but neither of them were able to explain why some arguments led to violence while others did not.

The team was struck by the humor both of them displayed when talking about anything other than violence. The team thought the arguments during the move would have been "sufficient to cause" violence in many couples. Mr. and Mrs. Harper's humor and practical jokes indicated to the team a way to be isomorphic and a way to promote cooperating. This latter was confirmed by the team's prediction, based on the couple's description, that their way of cooperating would include task performance. Therefore, the team prepared a "secret script" for a task that was a "practical joke," a key change for them to perform when they first got together in the evening (see Figure 4.6).

The team complimented them on having tried so many things to end the violence: moving to the city, shifting meal times, promises, self-control, and now therapy. Surely they must be frustrated by all this, and they must want a quick way to end the violence. But the team wondered if they would be satisfied with a method that just stopped the violence without ever finding out either "why did the violence happen" or "who is to blame for the violence." Mr. and Mrs. Harper agreed that stopping the violence was the primary thing. The con-

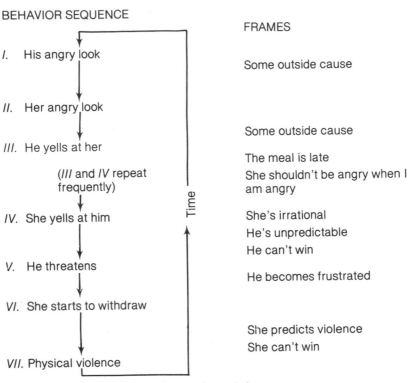

Figure 4.6.

ductor suggested that once the violence stopped, these answers might come.

The conductor then handed them the prepared notes, which were to be kept secret from the other person who would find out soon enough. They agreed.

1. Mr. Harper was instructed to come in the back door or to back in the front door when he was the least bit angry when he got home.
2. Mrs. Harper was asked to pick one dinner hour, no matter what she might think he wants. Further, she was asked to wait for him either in the kitchen or in the bathroom instead of at the front door if she was the least bit angry or she thought he might be angry.

They read the notes and agreed to give the ideas a try.

These clues were designed on the prediction that they would be able to find a way of cooperating with direct tasks and that they would find the results of these practical jokes to be humorous. Should either or both follow the clues, then the "getting home sequence" would be different enough, and the meeting would be in a different key. What exact behaviors might follow, the team could not predict. Nor were they naive enough to predict that this change of key would necessarily end the violence since there probably was more to the sequence and the frames around the events. But this approach might prevent violence between the first and the second sessions, which is the scope of first session interventions and predictions.

Session 2

Mr. and Mrs. Harper each tried the suggestions in the notes. When Mr. Harper backed in the front door a little earlier than Mrs. Harper expected him home, she burst out laughing and he quickly followed. Another day she was waiting in the bathroom when he came in the back door. She was surprised to find him waiting for her in the kitchen. Mrs. Harper had the meals each day 45 minutes after his usual time to come home.

In the past when violence occurred, it never happened in the kitchen, the bathroom, the basement, or outside the house. Violence often happened two or three times during a two-week period, and then it would not happen for several months. During these months they would still have arguments, but neither of them were clear about the differences between arguments that led to violence and those that did not. Nor were they able to describe how either type of argument came to an end. The only notable difference between arguments: Violent fights usually happened immediately after he got home, and nonviolent ones would start later in the evening.

To the team it seemed clear that either Mr. or Mrs. Harper might become angry at something "outside their relationship," and therefore the violence happened after they got together while "fighting mad"—a self-fulfilling prophecy. The team recalled that the most recent violence was brought to a halt when the phone rang. Therefore, the team suspected that some signal to end arguments might prove to be of use to the Harpers.

Based on their response report that was straightforward (column 1 of the decision tree), the team decided they could continue cooperating with the Harpers by giving another direct task. They were also aware that because of the Harpers' practical jokes and the response report, they could continue cooperating by suggesting practical jokes or other "illogical" gimmicks. The team also wanted to find out if there were "stop signs" involved in the nonviolent sequence that could be generalized to the violent sequence.

The team congratulated the Harpers on following what might have seemed to be silly instructions the week before. The conductor asked them to nod if, while doing these things or later, other equally silly ideas occurred to them. Both nodded. The conductor asked them to keep these practical jokes to themselves and to use these ideas next time the situation occurred. They agreed. The conductor also asked them to keep track of how any nonviolent arguments they had came to an end. Not how or if they resolved the issues, just how they were able to stop the argument. They agreed to this task.

The team predicted that the Harpers would use some more practical jokes and that they would attempt to find the stop signs for arguments. The silly ideas that occurred to the Harpers seemed to be some evidence that the key change might have been effective in "destroying the old sequence." This notion was given more strength by the behaviors the Harpers described as following the secret jokes the team planned.

Session 3

The Hapers reported that their two nonviolent arguments in two weeks had "just drifted off into something else." Both of these happened later in the evening. One day when Mrs. Harper expected Mr. Harper to come home angry, she went out and bought him his favorite beer and a rose. As it turned out, she was right. Mr. Harper came in the back door, found the beer and the rose with a note: "I love you." Mrs. Harper waited in the bathroom until she was sure he found these. They had a fun evening together.

It seemed obvious that the Harpers had moved outside their original frame. The key change had destroyed the old sequence. Again, the Harpers reported a straightforward response (column 1) to a direct task. Now the team needed to continue cooperating in such a way that the Harpers could stay outside the old frame since neither of them could be expected to control his or her daily meetings in this fashion forever. Since the Harpers remained dubious about their having solved the violence problem and because the sign (his coming home and showing anger that did not lead to violence had not yet happened), the team decided to design a "structured fight" that followed Goffman's guidelines and that included a signal for ending. The structure includes arbitrary starts and stops, exaggeration of patterns, and clear signals for the beginning and the termination. It is social since it involves both of them. The intervention is based on the sequence the Harpers described (Figure 4.6). Since the Harpers' manner of cooperating included task performance, this intervention could further the work begun by the key change.

Mr. and Mrs. Harper were complimented on their continued development and use of silly, creative ideas. The team also complimented them on using the distraction method for ending the most recent arguments, although there is one difficulty with distraction methods: The people might not just drift off into something else; the argument could just switch topics.

The conductor thought that their fights, particularly the violent ones, were too much like street fights. They agreed; they did not seem to have rules. The conductor suggested that a fight with rules, like boxing, might be more beneficial. They thought the idea of rules might be helpful. The conductor then gave them the following rules for fights that they were to use on two different evenings in the following two weeks. These fights were to take place immediately after Mr. Harper returned from work.

Rules

1. Toss a coin to determine who goes first.
2. Then, the winner gets to yell and scream about anything that comes to mind for 10 uninterrupted minutes;
3. while the loser just listens.
4. Then, the loser gets to yell and scream about anything, not necessarily in response to the winner's complaints;
5. while the winner just listens.
6. Then, a 10-minute silent break between "rounds" before repeating.
7. A kitchen timer with a loud bell was to be used to signal the end of each 10-minute segment or round.
8. These "boxing matches" were to take place in the kitchen.

The conductor cautioned them about the possibility that on some other night during the two weeks he was afraid they might have an old-fashioned street fight. He explained that falling back into old habits once or twice was a normal part of the change process. He suggested that these structured fights might be enough to prevent the old fights, but that they should not be too surprised if a real fight happened.

Follow-Up

Mr. and Mrs. Harper did not have a return of the old fights. They reported following through on the structured fights that they found to relieve their tensions. Once before the fourth session, Mr. Harper came home with an angry look on his face, but no argument and no violence followed. Six months later they reported using the structured fight once in a while just to relieve tension. There had been no violence.

Comment. Certainly, this therapy was more complex than "just changing the key," although that technique can be seen as destroying the pattern. The other interventions can be seen as "correcting the harmony" so that it fits the new sequence, and, therefore, the new sequence could function as a normal pattern.

CHAPTER 5

The Möbius Strip

SYSTEMIC CONFUSION

Before the development of the binocular theory of change, the concept of isomorphism was developed as a descriptive tool used to explain post hoc the design of interventions. Subsequently, the concept has been broadened for use as a prescriptive tool for guiding the therapist's efforts in promoting change by intervening from a different angle based on a description of the family patterns. This development led to the mapping techniques introduced in Chapter 3.

The decision tree introduced in Chapter 4 was developed, first, to organize the team's observations of the patterns of cooperating that families had shown and, then, to help the team decide what type of intervention would most likely continue the team's efforts toward cooperating. This chapter will deal with the use of column 4 of the decision tree: vague or confusing response reports.

In many ways column 4 of the decision tree is the product of an attempt to fit an anomaly into an existing conceptual scheme. The MRI brief therapy model (65, 67) does not offer a therapist clear guidelines either for the treatment of couples or families who show themselves unable to describe a concrete and specific goal for therapy or for therapy when each person of a family has a specific goal that would exclude the others' goals.

Erickson's "confusion technique" (35) is a trance-induction technique that develops from building confusion upon confusion until the subject is ready and able to accept a clear statement from the hypnotist. That is, Erickson takes his first principle of accepting what the client brings (confusion in this case) and utilizes that behavior to develop a trance-induction procedure or technique.

By analogy, the couple or family with mutually exclusive goals, or goals that it is unable to articulate, can be described as a "confused system" in that neither the people nor an observer can know where the family is going, or where it wants to go, or perhaps even what it is that is going on.

From this point of view, the problem presented to the therapist can be described as "the confusion." From this, an "implied goal" of ending the confusion can be developed. Thus, Erickson's technique can be broadened for use with confused systems (18, 20). That is, the family therapist can accept what the family system brings, that is, its unique manner of showing how it cooperates (the confused patterns). Then the therapist can utilize those patterns to develop isomorphic interventions by building confusion upon confusion until some sort of clarity is achieved.

Systemic confusion seems to take many different forms, all of which can be labeled as "vague" when the description is broadened to include the suprasystem. Confused subsystems, and some other subsystems, can be seen to show some sort of vague patterns and some sort of vague manners of cooperating that often leave therapists showing confusion. This chapter will describe the use of the concepts of cooperating and ismorphism as they are applied to vague family patterns.

The two case examples will describe the discontinuous change processes that two couples went through during therapy. ("Discontinuous change" is a label for a change process described as occurring "by leaps"; whereas "continuous change" is a label used to describe change processes observed to occur in a "step-by-step" fashion.) Both couples made sudden leaps or changes following an "isomorphic intervention," which resembles the Möbius strip, a pattern that folds back upon itself. Since isomorphic interventions are based on a description that is a mirror image (but from a different angle) of the family patterns, repeated use of Möbius-type interventions has allowed BFTC to study discontinuous change processes (see Figure 5.1).

In a multicausal, open system it is difficult to label "cause-effect" as: "event$_1$ caused event$_2$." This way is not sufficient to describe a circular chain of events. The discontinuous change process can be seen as a complex interac-

Figure 5.1. The Möbius strip.

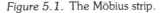
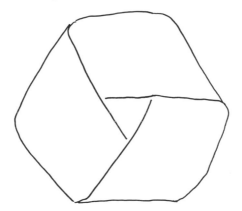

tion of various factors. Although in no particular order, these factors seem sa-
lient: the family's systemic confusion (as mapped by the therapist), the family's
demonstration of a vague manner of cooperating, the family's self-perceived
and described discomfort, the family's self-described fears of systemic disinte-
gration, and an intervention that is based on all of these factors that describes
the situation from a different angle. Each of these factors can be seen to interact
with each of the other factors separately and collectively, as seen in Figure 5.2.

THE PROTOTYPE

Early in the development of the brief family therapy model, shortly after
the invention of the consulting break and the perceived need for an ecosystemic perspective, but before the development of the binocular theory of
change, a couple came to BFTC for some help with its marriage. The initial
phone call was brief, and the information was mainly demographic.

In many ways the therapy with this couple was germinal to the development of the new model and the binocular theory of change. From the many reviews of the videotapes, the team eventually learned to *see* the couple's efforts
as attempts at cooperating rather than as a form of "resistance to change." During the first three sessions the team (de Shazer was conductor and Marilyn La-
Court was behind the mirror) designed tasks to help the couple become more
concrete and specific about its situation and what it wanted to see change. The
couple would respond in a way that seemed reasonable to it. From the couple's
point of view, its response was exactly what was called for by the task. How-

Figure 5.2.

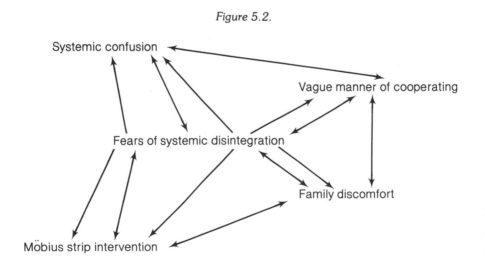

ever, the team was confused by the responses. Between sessions the team met several times to review tapes, and just prior to the fourth session an idea for an intervention was developed that was isomorphic with the couple's patterns and in line with the manner of cooperating it had shown.

When the team first designed the intervention, it was attempting to match the couple's particular use of the English language *and* the interactional nature of its complaints. Basically, the idea was that if the team could add even more confusion to the couple's patterns, then the couple might reverse its field, become less confused, and thus attempt to receive some clarity. This was based on a generalized version of the confusion technique (18, 20), but was rather experimental in this situation because the couple's type of systemic confusion was of a different type.

Before this "breakthrough" by the team, several hours of staff time were devoted to figuring out a way to help this couple become more concrete and specific. None of the suggestions proved useful. The team (and the BFTC staff) were victims of their own frame: that brief therapy needs to have a concrete and specific goal in order to be effective, a notion inherited from MRI. It was only when this particular set of patterns was described as "confused" that the team was able to use a confusion technique. This couple's therapy was before the development of the decision tree and, in fact, was part of what led to the designing of the tree and the inclusion of column 4.

Session 1

A sample of the couple's verbal exchange with the conductor in the first session:

DE SHAZER: What would you like to see change?

BARBARA: Get rid of a lot of shame that I seem to be carrying around with me. Get more self-confidence developed and become more, have more spontaneity and less tension. Get the tension out of me. *(Peter is watching closely, nodding.)* And, in our relationship, I'd like to get more freed up in my sexual expression with you [Peter], ah, my mind's gone blank.

DE SHAZER: Ah, OK.

BARBARA: I've got a lot thought up I'd really like to work on.

DE SHAZER: Obviously, we won't get it all in tonight anyway. So, when it comes back, that's the time to bring it up.

BARBARA: Sexual expression. I have a thing: I try to parent everybody, and I would like to be less of a parent to Peter. . . . Be more communicative than we have been. We've had some training, and that's improved everything, but I need to work on it more than I have been.

And, I really want to get out of this to be a better listener, particularly of Peter. That just goes across the board, I think.

DE SHAZER: Ah, that's a pretty good picture. How about you, Peter?

PETER: Well, for me, it's increasing my confidence level to kind of develop or heighten my ability to accept responsibility for myself and behaviors. I tend to pass the buck, or blame situations on other people for my inactivity, or my lack of response. I think that is one of the real big hang-ups. I think—what Barbara said, sexual expression—freeing myself up to allow myself the pleasures, or to be in the here and now versus thinking about situations before they occur, or setting things up in rigid analytical thinking. Kind of putting aside my ego. Just accepting myself.

DE SHAZER: OK.

BARBARA: *(Overlapping.)* Are you done? A very big one for me is accepting self-responsibility.

DE SHAZER: Well, what prompted you to call last week? Why then and not, say, six weeks ago?

BARBARA: Well, it's been put off. Procrastination. I keep thinking—each of us thinking—well, if we just work at it, use our communication skills, we should be able to handle it. I don't know what happened last week. I really got down in the pits again.

PETER: I think it was, for me, increased irritability. Just kind of heightening to the point of being fed up with the way things were going. Our conversation being irritable to each other. My losing patience and kind of pulling out. And, Barb getting down in the pits and depressed. To me, that was kind of the height, and I said, "Maybe we should."

BARBARA: I just kind of got pretty scared of, ah, just how I feel? Which feels pretty hopeless. *(Tears.)*

DE SHAZER: What's so hopeless? *(Scratching his head.)*

BARBARA: Just me, and that I'm a worthwhile human being?

PETER: When Barb's like that, I find myself backing out of the relationship.

DE SHAZER: *(Looking puzzled.)* After you back out, how do you get back in?

PETER: At times like that, I get a hold of myself, realize what I'm doing. Or, sometimes when Barb breaks down and cries, or says she needs some closeness, or whatever.

The conductor then attempted to clarify some of the above statements about the problem and tried to get some specific information that was buried in the above descriptions. However, these efforts met with little success. The couple's responses to these questions were similar to the above dialogue. Eventually, from watching the tapes (of this session and the next) the team learned some of the sequence: For some unknown reason Barbara would get "depressed," then Peter would try to cheer her up in a playful manner. She did not like what she called his "little-boy act," and so his attempt would further depress her, and then he would "back out."

The only concrete material to come out of the first three sessions was that Peter was rebuilding a valuable antique. Through very careful questions, it was discovered that Peter had been working on this project for years. Lately, he did very little work on it. This "gnawed" at Barbara because it was their plan to sell the antique to finance a move to another part of the country. So, periodically she would nag about it, but he still would not do anything. Barbara saw this as a big worry since she really did want to move. In fact, she was afraid Peter would never finish it and, therefore, they would never move. Peter said he did not work on it because he was afraid the move would not live up to their expectations, even though he saw the move as probably helping him reach his real "potential." Therefore, it was safe for him not to work on the project and face the possibility of losing this dream.

At this point in the first session, the team took its consulting break. The data around the antique were the only specific material developed in the first 40 minutes of the session. This type of systemic confusion paralyzed Barbara and Peter and left both of them to wonder about what it is that is going on. But finishing the antique was the only concrete item they both agreed about that the team could think of as a goal. However, the team decided not to pursure the matter actively because it wished to avoid seeming to be on "her side" by picking this as a formal goal. Although Barbara and Peter both said they wanted to move, when and where was very vague. Again, this seemed more "her goal" than his. The team decided to make further attempts at goal definition.

When the conductor returned to the session, he asked the couple to think about how they would know for sure that therapy had been successful. They thought this a good idea, and the session ended. The team predicted Barbara and Peter would return for the subsequent session.

Session 2

The couple's response to this task centered around several issues: (1) the need for unconditional love, (2) the question of how to know what is "really real," and (3) the couple's feelings of being trapped into trying to please. Once these issues were resolved, they thought they would then know that therapy had been successful. However, the conductor was unable to get Barbara and Peter to describe how they would *know* these three issues were resolved, or what would be different about their behaviors, or their lives in general once these issues were resolved. They would "just know, and feel better."

The team attempted to develop a task that was closer to the couple's language and world view. The conductor asked them to think about how they would know for sure that they each were really loved by the other. "What behaviors would you see that would let you know this issue is starting to get resolved?" As a parting work, this question was phoned in: "How's project antique?" Peter had not worked on it at all.

Session 3

Peter announced to the team (behind the mirror) that he had worked for 10 hours on the antique while Barbara was out of town. He had been neither reminded or nagged by Barbara and did the work on his own initiative. They both agreed that when Barbara had been home, things were less tense. She had not felt sad or depressed, and he did not feel a need to back out. It also turned out that they had had sexual intercourse for the first time in five months, a topic to which they alluded in the first session but avoided afterward. They had both thought about the task, but neither of them was able to come up with any specific behavioral signs. Each would "just know" for sure that he or she was really loved by the other.

During the consulting break the team decided that the previous task had also been "off target." Although the couple did the task in a straight-forward manner the team was still blinded by looking for concrete and specific behaviors. The team decided to attempt a task that included the necessity for some action. The team was aware that "something was different" and that Barbara and Peter had made some changes: less sadness, less backing out, and more sexual activity. However, the team was less than sure that these changes were "differences that made a difference." That is, the team did not know if these changes were in the old frame or were steps outside the old frame. Since the entire session seemed more clear, the team decided that these changes interconnected with the therapy. And even if this assumption were to turn out to be wrong, it decided to act "as if" the differences were due to therapy since Barbara and Peter did make some shifts since the start of therapy that might be built upon.

DE SHAZER: We are a bit concerned with just how fast things seemed to have changed in your situation. For the better part of two weeks, you have not felt sad or depressed, and you have not had to back out or attempt to cheer her up. We worry when things change that fast because then the slightest little setback looks so damn big that people are tempted to think "it's back to the way it was." So, watch out. Slow it down somehow.

Between now and next session, we would like for each of you to initiate some new, joint activity. It does not need to be fancy, or cost a lot of money. It can be anything, even something silly. Don't talk about it, or let the other know "this is it!" Let's see if the other can figure it out.

Session 4

When Barbara and Peter returned for the next session two weeks later, they reported that the "improvement" had continued for a few days. But then, things went back to usual when she became sad again. He tried to cheer her up, and the pattern continued. They both reported trying to think of something new for them to do, but only Peter claimed to have figured something out and to have initiated it. His report surprised Barbara since she thought he had initiated *two* different things. Barbara was displeased with herself because she had been unable to think of anything to initiate. In turn, Barbara's report surprised Peter because he had perceived her as initiating something. (Therefore, she could be seen as having done the task without realizing it.) Peter had initiated going bowling (which they had not done in many years), while Barbara initiated a game of Monopoly (which they had never played by themselves).

The main theme of the session centered around one major question: "How do I know what is really real?" When things went bad, each doubted that the other person really loved him or her unconditionally. And, Barbara's task performance/nonperformance brought this question into further doubt: How could he have perceived that she did the task when she herself thought she did not? (This task performance issue is another example of the systemic confusion.)

At the end of the session the conductor presented a planned intervention, which the team designed between sessions. The intervention is closely patterned on Barbara and Peter's interactional and communicational style.

DE SHAZER: You know, your sadness serves another purpose. It's not just self-protective. It protects him too.

BARBARA: *(Nodding.)* I had not thought of it that way

DE SHAZER: It protects him in several ways. One of the things it does is, he's going to try to cheer you up. It protects him from—If it wasn't there he'd have to commit himself to believing that you seriously do love him.

BARBARA: I hadn't looked at it like that.

DE SHAZER: And the same for your playfulness. It protects her—as far as we can tell—from having to face the fact that you really do love her.

And, therefore, she'd have to commit herself to believing in the reality of your love.

So, the playfulness and the sadness work out pretty well. And, there's nothing wrong with being either playful or sad. Now, we think you both should continue to be sad or playful as the need may be.
(Both were observed to be nodding throughout this message.)

Comment. In the first four sessions, Barbara has described seeing her sadness as self-protective. When she was sad, she would not reach out for Peter, and, therefore, she saw herself as not having to risk being rejected. She saw Peter's playfulness as self-protective since he prevented himself from having to face "negative emotions." She complained about his playfulness since it "caused" her to become more sad; and he complained about her sadness since it "caused" them to become more and more distant.

The above rather confusing intervention was based on a development of Erickson's confusion technique as it was expanded from hypnotherapy into the family therapy arena (18). In general, when using this type of intervention, the conductor can employ a barrage of words within a shifting frame of reference or ambiguity. The context can be shifted to create a lack of referential index that prevents the people from concentrating on the details of the conductor's verbal output. The couple's need to focus, or find meaning, is further and further frustrated *until they rebel* and demand clarity. Once introduced, the conductor will approach later sessions with the same sort of ambiguity and confusion.

When the team developed this intervention between the third and fourth sessions, the phrasing of the message was just designed to "confuse" Barbara and Peter by *reframing their complaints about each other as mutually beneficial.* The attempt to reframe both complaints interactionally was part of the attempt to confuse things further so that Barbara and Peter might respond with some clarity.

Later Sessions

Three weeks later Barbara and Peter returned. Peter reported that less than 10 hours of work remained on the antique. They reported that their sex life had continued to improve, and the frequency had increased. Both of them reported less tension, although neither of them could point to a reason for these changes. At one point the conductor made a very ambiguous statement, and Barbara asked him to be more specific. In general, Barbara and Peter seemed more relaxed and less confused. He reported taking a firm stand on an issue at work that gave him some satisfaction, and she was pleased that the antique was nearly finished.

It was not until the final session, one month later, that the real clarity became obvious to the team through Barbara and Peter's exchanges with the conductor. (The team had asked several other BFTC staff to join it for this session in case the original confusion had returned.) During the session, Barbara and Peter were much more concise. The antique was finished and up for sale. They had set a deadline for the move, and he had taken a job-hunting trip. He found a position that suited him. Further, they had decided she should become pregnant as soon as the move was completed. Prior to this session, all of these decisions were "out there in the future," to be decided "one day." By mutual agreement, the session ended in a half-hour, and therapy was terminated.

There did indeed seem to be a "difference that made a difference" in the observed interactions between Barbara and Peter and between them and the conductor. The extra members of the team who observed the final session had viewed the tapes, and they too observed a tremendous difference between the first session and the final session.

●   ●   ●

The BFTC staff subsequently reviewed the tapes in hopes of achieving more clarity about the effectiveness of the intervention. The team was not quite satisfied that it was a simple matter, first, of giving the couple back its confusion, then, watching the couple rebel, and then, seeing the couple become more clear. A more rigorous explanation was sought: Previous uses of a confusion technique often produced similar results, and so the simple explanation satisfied. This case presented a unique opportunity to develop some understanding of the application of the technique and the particular construction of this intervention.

As the team reviewed the tapes, the couple's confusion—if anything—became more clear: That is, it was *more confusing* to the team. Barbara and Peter's language was filled with incongruities, ambiguities, fuzzy functions; and their sentences were often ill-formed, including a lack of referential index (2, 3). In general, these linguistic phenomena are thought of as "individual" in nature not as "systemic." However, watching the tapes helped the team to learn the systemic nature of these linguistic difficulties. Peter and Barbara might be described as sharing a unique grammar that each seemed to think he or she understood and each seemed to think the other understood. As the BFTC staff listened to their conversations, it heard one phrase that lacked referential index piled upon another. Therefore, it was no longer surprising to the staff that the team had become confused because there often was no way for the listener to determine "by context" what some vague word or phrase actually meant. It began to be clear to the team that Barbara and Peter could not make decisions because they only *assumed* that the other person did really understand and this assumption seemed faulty. The team at last understood that Barbara and Peter were being as clear as they could be about their problems, which neither of them understood in the least.

Although the opening speeches (presented verbatim above) were confusing to the team, Barbara and Peter indicated to the team that they fully understood what the other was saying. However, various sequences in the tapes were filled with even more ambiguities, and further reviewing gave the team the strong impression that Barbara and Peter *mistakenly* assumed that the other understood.

More importantly, it became clear to the team that Barbara and Peter were not "resisting." Instead, the team saw clearly that Barbara and Peter were trying very hard to let the team know what they wanted from therapy. The team did not really find a way of cooperating until the fourth session, although the conductor had quickly adopted a vague and ambiguous type of speech in the first session. But once the team found a way of cooperating with the couple's way of cooperating, the couple received the bonus of a perceptual shift, as demonstrated by the changes in behavior.

The reviews of the intervention in the fourth session clarified for the team which aspects seem to have made the rather confusing intervention as effective as it seems to have been. The intervention was isomorphic but from a different angle that reframed both individual complaints into interactional or mutual complaints. The "sad-playful" sequence, punctuated in this fashion, provided the team with a description that was the interactional foundation for the intervention, as illustrated in Figure 5.3.

Because of Barbara's frame, she saw her sadness as self-protective and Peter's playfulness as self-protective while also being aggravating to her. On the

Figure 5.3.

MUTUAL REACTION SEQUENCE

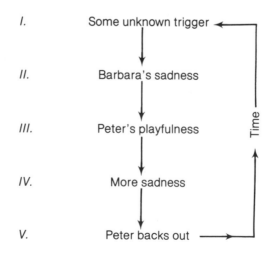

other hand, Peter saw her sadness as self-protective and aggravating to him, and he saw his backing out as also aggravating to her.

The intervention reframed the whole protection idea (attributed to the arrows in Figure 5.3 between *III* and *II* and between *IV* and *III*) to emphasize the mutuality or the circularity. Therefore, the protection (from this new angle) became "other-protective" rather than self-protective. That is, the Möbius intervention described Barbara's complaints about Peter as actually protective of her, while Peter's complaints about Barbara were actually protective of him.

The Möbius intervention described the sequence as serving a specific purpose in their relationship. The mutual protection was described as protecting each of them from knowing that the other did indeed love unconditionally. This assurance of the "reality" of the other's love was something they both desired and was a much discussed topic. Therefore, the Möbius intervention turned back on itself and described their main complaints about each other (now labeled as "protective of the other") as serving to protect the other from reaching a much desired goal.

From the study of this intervention prototype, BFTC learned a lot about how families show their attempts to cooperate in their own unique fashion. Further, the team learned more about how to promote team-family cooperating. From the Möbius intervention, we learned more about the usefulness of isomorphic interventions. From the map of this intervention (Figure 5.4), the team can develop similar interventions when the couple's complaints form part of a mutual reaction sequence of behavior.

With maps of this sort (Figures 5.3 and 5.4), the therapist can be prepared to design other interventions to use when similar maps are developed as descriptions of couples' interactions. The Möbius map seems useful in guiding the therapist's intervention design with couples who have complaints about each other that are related steps in a sequence. On the map in Figure 5.4, "A" stands for one person at a time, and the other person's ("B") complaints are treated separately: The map is used twice to design the intervention. The pair of complaints needs to be "interactional and sequential"; that is, Peter can be described as playful "in response" to Barbara's sadness. Further, the complaints need to be framed by the couple as "mutually causitive"; that is, Peter saw his playfulness as "caused by" Barbara's sadness, while Barbara saw her increased sadness as "caused by" Peter's playfulness. These points seem to be important considerations in the use of the Möbius map because the described interaction pattern that serves as a foundation defines the structure of the map. If the mutual complaints—with or without the systemic confusion—are spaced out in time or are seen as parts of different sequences, then these territories need a different map.

The use of these maps with another case will provide further clarification of the Möbius map's usefulness as a prescriptive tool for designing interventions

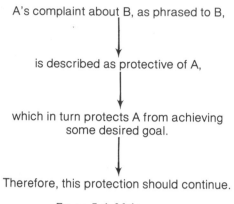

A's complaint about B, as phrased to B,

is described as protective of A,

which in turn protects A from achieving
some desired goal.

Therefore, this protection should continue.

Figure 5.4. Möbius map.

with couples who have mutual complaints. Since the couple's response report also describes a discontinuous change, there are interesting conclusions to be drawn from the processes involved.

A SECOND CASE EXAMPLE

Meg and Tony Cummings had been married for 19 years and had four children all under 16 years old. At the time of the first session, they had been separated for six months. After four and one-half months they started dating each other, while other contact remained limited. These dates had been fun for both of them until Tony started to talk about coming home. This topic started to occur two and one-half weeks before the first session. This topic made Meg feel tense, and her tension prompted Tony to start feeling "desperate" about the situation. He wondered if she really did care and if she was really interested in getting back together.

Tony's work often took him away from home for days at a time, which he did not like; but he liked the job itself. When he was at work, he frequently called Meg. These calls irritated Meg since she thought he was checking up on her, whereas he thought he was just trying to let her know about his interest in her. These calls were one of the triggers for the many arguments they had had over the years. Since they both described themselves as stubborn, their fights could last for up to five days, after which they frequently went for weeks without speaking to each other. As near as either of them could remember, this was the 12th separation in their marriage. It was the longest and the most serious. Meg had gone so far this time as to consider a divorce and to see a lawyer. However, neither of them *really* wanted a divorce since they both said they loved each other.

Session 1

Meg and Tony's goal was clearly stated: They wanted to get back together *and* to stay together. At this point, they had no specific timetable in mind. Meg felt that a very positive step toward their goal would be when she felt comfortable having Tony visit the house. For Tony, a very positive step would be when Meg gave him a show of affection—a simple hug—without his having to ask for it.

Meg and Tony were seen in a setting without a mirror and without a team. de Shazer was the therapist. This BFTC branch office was set up to test out the methodology involved in using this new model and format when working as a solo therapist.

Once the signs and goals were established, the therapist took a break to "think about what you have told me so far." It seemed clear that both Meg and Tony desired to get back together and that they had already started to work on this project. However, they had split up many times before, and they had found ways to get back together without the help of any therapist. Therefore, the problem was not getting them back together, but somehow making this re-unification different in a way that might allow them to stay together.

Since they had already taken steps along the path of getting back together, the therapist's task was to cooperate with them along this chosen route. The steps they already took formed the base of the compliment and, therefore, helped the therapist design an intervention that was isomorphic. The therapist was aware that Meg and Tony might decide not to reunite, but if they did, then there would likely be yet another argument and perhaps another split. This seemed their usual pattern.

When the therapist returned from his break, he gave them the following intervention, which he had written down for himself:

> DE SHAZER: It seems to me that it takes a lot of guts for the two of you to decide to work together on getting back together. I'm impressed with that. I don't know what the odds are on your getting back together and then staying together. And, I'm sure you don't either, and I'm impressed that you are willing to try nonetheless.
>
> Now, it seems to me that you've made the first steps: dating, talking about getting back together, and now coming here. These all seem in the right direction, and these steps seem appropriately spaced and I agree, you should continue to go slow.
>
> Between now and next time we meet, I want each of you—

separately—to think about what you do not want to see change about your relationship.

TONY: I see. That will give us something positive to build on.

DE SHAZER: Yeah, and you might want to take notes.

The session ended at that point. Both agreed to "continue to go slowly," and both agreed to do the task.

Meg and Tony seemed to pay close attention to both phases of the intervention. Both nodded at several points, and both seemed relaxed and cheerful at the end of the session. The therapist predicted that they would return for the next session and that both would do something in line with the task that would provide further information about their manner of cooperating. Meg seemed particularly relieved when the therapist agreed they "go slow," but the therapist was not sure about Tony's reaction. The therapist did not expect any significant changes during the interval, although he did expect some reports of "more steps."

Session 2

Three weeks later, Tony had been home for over a week.

DE SHAZER: Well, how did that happen?

MEG: One night we just decided to try again. Tony was more sure than me, but I was comfortable enough to let him stay.

DE SHAZER: Hmmm. I worry about that. It seems like you two are really rushing things. I hope that doesn't mean it'll come apart as fast as it went back together.

TONY: Since then we both have been trying hard to be nice to each other.

Since the first part of their goal had been met, they decided to work on their arguments, which they saw as driving them apart in the first place. Without these fights, they both felt they could stay together. They reported that since Tony moved back in they had five really good days and only one bad day. They had a small argument that was quickly over. They made sure they did not allow themselves to go to bed mad, which was a new rule for them. Meg thought that they could manage to say together if this became a regular pattern with them.

They described their typical fight sequence: (1) Meg would be silent (for some reason). (2) Tony would interpret this as "she's in a bad mood," which prompted him to try to find out "why." Then (3) she would answer "nothing." (4) But this would not satisfy him, so he would continue asking questions. (5) She would ask him to leave her alone, and (6) if he did not leave her alone, then they would have an argument. That is, her silences were seen as "causing" him to ask questions, while his questions were seen as "causing" her to be more silent.

In response to the previous session's task, Meg saw that she did not want Tony to change his sense of humor or his thorough approach to challenges. She also did not want him to stop being sympathetic and understanding with people. She saw him as patient and sociable, which she did not want to see change.

Tony did not want to lose the good times they had when they were away from the children. Furthermore, he did not want to change the fact that Meg was honest, thoughtful, and faithful. He also liked her persistance. (This was a slight modification of the task that asked them to deal with their relationship, *not* the other's personality. Therefore, a subsequent task should allow room for any modification.)

Their description of their typical sequence that led up to an argument bears a striking resemblance to the "mutual reaction sequence" in the previous example, and a similar map, shown in Figure 5.5, was constructed. This map of Meg and Tony's pattern led the therapist to start considering the possibility of using the Möbius map to design the intervention in some subsequent session,

Figure 5.5.

MUTUAL REACTION SEQUENCE

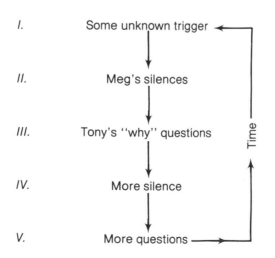

which might be an intervention isomorphic enough to promote some significant changes.

Since Meg and Tony were back together, the first part of their goal was
met. However, this did not seem like a move outside their frame, just a move
within. It did not change the frame, and, therefore, the likelihood was that they
would split up again. Developing ways to argue that did not leave them angry at
bedtime seemed a reasonable enough sign to attach to the second part of their
goal—staying together. The therapist was not clear about the signal Meg and
Tony used to end the arguments, particularly those they ended without any
clear rationale.

> DE SHAZER: I'm impressed with all the changes you two have made in the
> past three weeks. It seems you've worked hard on getting back to-
> gether and on being nice to each other. I'm sure that avoiding argu-
> ments has not been easy, but you've done it. One small fight in a
> week is quite good, particularly since neither of you went to bed mad.
>
> However, I worry about how fast things have changed. It seems
> to me that if you had one argument that ended up with either of you
> still mad at bedtime, well, then you'd think it was the "same old
> thing," and you might split up again.
>
> As much as you both would like the fights to stop, that's not likely
> in the immediate future. People who live together are going to disa-
> gree now and then. So, what I'd like you both to do between now and
> next time is to watch how these arguments or disagreements cease—
> how you get them to stop, or at least to end a particular round. Just
> note it down for me.
>
> TONY: You mean, you'd like to know what happens after the fights?
>
> DE SHAZER: Right. I'd like to know what each of you do so that you do not
> go to bed mad at each other.
>
> MEG: I see. And you want us to write it down.

This task is easily modifiable: They could not write the reasons down, or
they could only pay attention to the fights that did not cause them to go to bed
mad, or they could pay attention to the fights that they could not stop and so
caused them to go to bed angry. The therapist predicted that they would be
able to note *some* of "how" their arguments stopped. Further, he predicted that
they would have a big fight, but they would not be able to report how this one
stopped. He also predicted that, for the most part, Meg and Tony would have a
good two weeks. Since the therapist told them to go slowly about getting back
together, and they got together rather quickly, the therapist could also predict
some likelihood that Meg and Tony would be unable to do the homework
because of a lack of arguments to report about.

Session 3

Two weeks later, Meg called to cancel the session because Tony had to work. Meg reported that everything was great between them. Various appointments were canceled with the same "great" report until the third session was finally held 12 weeks after the second.

When Meg and Tony arrived for the session, they were in the middle of a disagreement. They were both off work, and this dispute had started 10 hours earlier. They reported that during the previous 12 weeks, they had only a couple of very small fights, but neither of them remembered how they had ceased.

> MEG: If he'd only accept me as I am, then none of this would matter.
>
> TONY: But you keep changing your moods. I never know where I stand with you, because when you're silent, I keep wondering, "What did I do?"
>
> MEG: And, I keep telling you that you didn't do anything, I just need time alone, quiet time.
>
> TONY: But I always think you're mad, and . . .
>
> MEG: (Overlapping.) But, I'm just tired.

Tony described needing to be reassured constantly that Meg loved him and was not angry, and he became "jealous" of any other interest Meg showed. He saw her silences as preoccupation with someone or something else. When he questioned her about loving him, she started again to wish he were out of the house. However, she continued to try to avoid fights by being silent, which served further to "provoke" his questions.

Tony described her silences as "mood swings," and therefore he would nag her about these, trying to get to the bottom of it. He continued to think that each and every silence was a signal that she was angry at him for something he did.

The therapist, who knew that the next session was as likely to be postponed as not, decided to end the session without any explicit task, just with a compliment. And the therapist decided to have a written intervention ready for the next session, one based on their mutual reaction sequence. At this point, reframing the status quo without calling it either a fight or an argument was in keeping with the plan, although the temptation was to give the same assignment. However, a long interval between sessions might make this an ineffective clue, even if they should report doing it. Of course, their response report also indicated that they did not do the task, and column 5 in Figure 4.3 suggests "no concrete task should now be given."

> DE SHAZER: I'm really impressed with the ability you two have to hang in there, to stick with trying to solve this problem. As much as I, too,

think it would be desirable to accept each other just as you are, I don't
suspect that's going to be easy or quick. I suspect that you both will
continue to, Meg and Tony avoid fights—as best you can.

TONY: But what should we do?

MEG: This can't go on this way.

DE SHAZER: Well, I don't know. It seems more complicated than I first
thought. I need to think about this. I guess you need to just hang in
there.

TONY: But, what about her mood swings?

MEG: What about his jealousy?

DE SHAZER: Right now, that's confusing me. I need to talk with my group
about it.

The therapist predicted either (1) this disagreement would become a fight
and they would split or (2) for some unexplained reason, things would suddenly become much better, similar to what happened after the first two sessions. If
the first prediction proved correct, the therapist thought the split would be
short.

Between sessions the therapist designed an intervention based on the
Möbius map. Meg's complaint about Tony directly followed his complaint
about her. Her silences were described as causing his questions, while his question "caused" her to become more silent. The isomorphism between Meg and
Tony's complaint patterns and Barbara and Peter's complaint patterns, plus the
erratic and therefore vague and confused scheduling that confused the effectiveness of the tasks and their response reports, all gave rise to the idea that an
intervention designed on the Möbius map might be effective. As the therapist
reviewed the case and started to design an intervention, it became clear that
Meg and Tony's mutual reaction sequence could be mapped onto the mutual
reaction sequence of the previous example. In both cases, the initial trigger described for the sequence is "unknown," and in both cases, this trigger is followed by the two complaints in step fashion, one right behind the other.

Session 4

This session followed the third by a month. Meg and Tony reported that
"things are going well." They had fewer than one argument per week during
the month. Tony reported that Meg did not brood during the entire period.

MEG: Just showing him that I love him more often seems to make for less
conflict.

TONY: My jealousy is getting better because she's showing affection more
than ever before.

The temptation at this point is to abort the planned intervention since the mutual reaction sequence does not seem to have been in operation. Meg and Tony seem to have met their signs and to be on the road to their goal of staying together. However, their larger pattern seems to include these periods of peace, and the therapist decided that Meg and Tony could be helped to stay outside their old frame, which now seemed cracked if not broken. Perhaps intervening about the mutual reaction sequence during a period of peace might prove more effective. It might change things enough, if it has the predicted outcome, to help them stay outside of their old frame.

After the break, the therapist read the following message:

DE SHAZER: I've talked to our consultant—a psychiatrist—and to the rest of my group about your situation. We've come to several conclusions. I'm not sure I agree with it all.

I'm glad you pointed out to me on the phone when you canceled two weeks ago that I seem to have been sidestepping the jealousy issue and the mood swings. Sometimes that happens. Perhaps I've been remiss. My only excuse is that I feel these issues are so central.

It seems to us that Meg becomes silent when she has heard too many things. We suspect that she has very sensitive ears, and when there's been too many words, too much noise, she turns off her ears. It doesn't matter what the noise is: words, music, car horns, etc.

On the other hand, Tony becomes upset when he sees things out of place. We suspect he has sensitive eyes, and he sees "red" when there's too much mess and confusion. When Tony sees too many things out of place, his eyes become tired of working and he becomes upset.

We suspect that somewhere along the line—perhaps while growing up—Tony learned that "silence equals anger." Maybe your mother made you be quiet when she was mad at you. And, of course, you were mad at her. Therefore, being silent means being mad.

Now, that's not all there is to it. It's not that simple. We think the jealousy and the mood swings are very important parts of your relationship. I had hoped I could help you two get along better, keep your marriage together, without messing this up. Because I see the silences and the jealousy as very central. We suspect that you're going to find this a bit of a puzzle. So do I. So, let me finish reading this before you comment.

It seems to us, Tony, that your jealousy protects Meg from discovering just how much she cares for you, Tony. Your jealousy assures her that you care. She reacts with mood swings and silences because, if she did not, she's afraid you would be overwhelmed by the depth of her feelings.

It seems to us, Meg, that your silences further protect Tony from realizing how constant your feelings really are. If he were to realize how faithful and true your feelings are for him, then he'd not have the challenge which he needs. He might become bored—or even depressed—if he didn't have the challenges your silences present him.

Therefore, we think you two need to continue to protect each other with your jealousy and your silences. Meg, you need to be silent whenever you feel Tony needs a challenge or that he might be overwhelmed. And Tony, you need to be jealous whenever you think Meg doesn't know you care, or you're getting bored.

The therapist observed each of them nodding at various times while he was reading the message. He said that he would mail them copies and suggested they should think about this prior to the following session, which was scheduled to be in one month.

The therapist predicted this intervention would help Meg and Tony stay outside of their old frame and thus continue to make changes that might even be discontinuous. He further predicted there would be "no big fights" and that complaints about either jealousy or mood swings would be minimal.

Follow-Up

One week later, Tony called to cancel the next session because he knew in advance that he was going to be unavailable. He reported—without being asked—that things were pretty confusing, but that he no longer felt jealous and had not noticed Meg having mood swings. He rescheduled. A week prior to the rescheduled session, Meg called to say that everything was fine and they no longer needed therapy. A further report was received from the referral source, a close friend of the family who had known them for 15 years: He had never seen them enjoy themselves as much as they did now. "It's hard to imagine they're the same couple. They don't fight anymore." A call some months later received the same report from Meg.

ISOMORPHISM

The behavioral sequence in both case studies presented here can be mapped together (see Figure 5.6). The isomorphism between the two complaint patterns provides a bonus for the therapist and the team because the two different case studies provide different points of view that create ideas about systems.

What is striking is that the Möbius strip interventions map can be used to

BEHAVIOR SEQUENCE

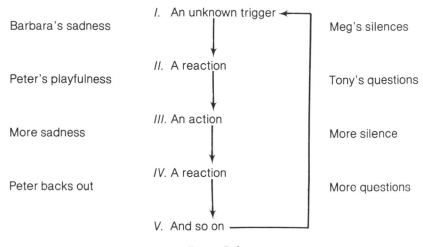

Figure 5.6.

describe the interventions in both cases and that these maps can be combined as shown in Figure 5.7.

Of course, the first case was a prototype for the second case and various other cases. However, the isomorphism obtained between the two maps and the similarity of the couples' reported responses are striking. Both couples seemed to go through a period of increased confusion while the complaints diminished, and then suddenly (at least it is sudden from the observer's point of view) they made big changes. The Cummings' family friend "hardly knew they were the same people." Both couples can be seen to have reorganized without their old complaint patterns. In short, the systemic confusion/vagueness seems to have disappeared.

There seems to be some interconnective link between the Möbius intervention and the changes that followed. The binocular theory of change suggests that the sequence after the intervention can now be seen by the couples from a different angle. That is, if the sequence should appear to be starting, various elements of the names of the context are "slippery" enough (i.e., have started to develop a different attributed meaning) that a new sequence can develop spontaneously. For instance, should Barbara become "sad" again (which is likely), Peter is apt to wonder if he should "protect her by becoming playful." There is some probability that the meaning of his playfulness and/or her sadness is slippery enough that a different behavior might be prompted. In

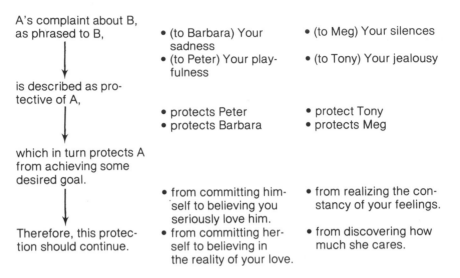

A's complaint about B, as phrased to B,

↓

is described as protective of A,

↓

which in turn protects A from achieving some desired goal.

↓

Therefore, this protection should continue.

- (to Barbara) Your sadness
- (to Peter) Your playfulness

- protects Peter
- protects Barbara

- from committing himself to believing you seriously love him.
- from committing herself to believing in the reality of your love.

- (to Meg) Your silences
- (to Tony) Your jealousy

- protect Tony
- protects Meg

- from realizing the constancy of your feelings.
- from discovering how much she cares.

Figure 5.7. Möbius strip intervention.

fact, Barbara did become "sad" during the interval prior to the last session. Peter, instead of becoming playful, put his arms around her and listened for an hour. They then made the decision to have a child as soon as their move was completed.

Although we have no knowledge of this, there is some probability that should Peter have responded to her sadness with playfulness, then Barbara might wonder if she should "protect him by becoming more sad." There is some chance that this meaning is also slippery enough to prompt a different response from Barbara. For instance, she might respond with some playful behavior of her own or she might become openly angry. Either would start a new sequence. The intervention introduced the possibility of some random behavior from a class of behaviors not included in the original sequence. What that specific behavior (or specific behaviors) might be is impossible to predict.

CHAPTER 6
Goals: Balance Theoretical Maps*

BALANCE THEORY

Although the use of balance theory for describing family relationships and change has been discarded as epistemologically flawed (see Chapter 1), Heider's theory (41) can be a helpful tool for guiding our thinking about the goal directedness of therapy (21). Heider describes the relationships (A to B, B to C, C to A) among three elements (A, B, C) of a configuration (or mental set) as interdependent-with-each-other relationship. These relationships are described as naturally tending toward a balanced state (a stable state), and once in a balanced state configurations tend to remain that way. Heider defined two types of balance: "In the case of three entities, a balanced state exists if all three relations are positive . . . or if two are negative and one positive" (41, p. 110). Furthermore, "if no balanced state exists, then forces toward this state will arise" (41, p. 108). If a configuration is balanced in either of the two ways, it will tend to remain balanced. However, if the configuration is not balanced, it will tend to move toward *either* of the two balanced states: (*1*) all relations positive or (*2*) two negative relations and one positive relation.

A brief illustration using the signed-diagraphs developed by Cartwright and Harary (14) will clarify Heider's theory. For the sake of simplicity, the illustration will be presented from one person's point of view as Heider originally conceived the theory.

If an individual, say "*p*," is involved with another individual, say "*o*," whom he loves and *p* makes a ceramic pot, say "*x*," that he really likes, then it is important to *p* that *o* also likes *x*. If indeed *o* does like *x*, then the configuration is balanced, a state that can be mapped (as shown in Figure 6.1, graph *1*).

If *o* does not like *x*, then *p* is described to be in a tense situation. The configuration, or *p*'s cognitive map of the situation, is not balanced: two positive relations and one negative (see graph *2*). According to Heider's theory, within

*Another version of some of the material in this chapter previously appeared as "On Transforming Symptoms: An Approach to an Erickson Procedure," *American Journal of Clinical Hypnosis* **22**: 17-28, 1979.

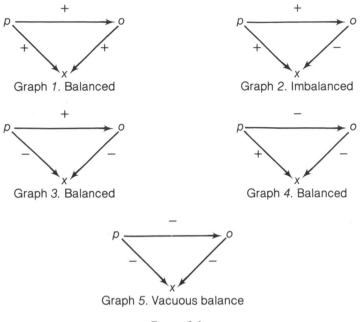

Figure 6.1.

this configuration there will be tendencies to shift toward a balanced state; (1) o can be seen by p to start liking x (graph 1); (2) p can shift to disliking x (graph 3); (3) p can shift to disliking o (graph 4); or, if worse comes to worse, (4) p can shift to disliking both o and x (graph 5). Graph 5 illustrates a special case called "vacuous balance" (14) in which all relations are described as negative, a configuration that tends to endure and is, therefore, considered to be balanced in a vacuous manner.

Cartwright and Harary (14) generalized Heider's theory for use with groups or units of any number and further expanded the theory to include both reciprocal (symmetrical) and nonreciprocal (complementary) relationships. Essentially, the same measures of balance are used: A balanced state is seen to exist if either (1) all relations are described as positive or (2) the observer describes an even number of negative relations. Vacuous balance is seen to exist if all relations described by the observer are labeled "negative."

With balance theory as a descriptive tool, an explication of one of Erickson's procedures will illustrate the goal directedness of his approach. The Erickson procedure will be mapped using balance theory, and then this map will be further developed to illustrate the goal directedness of brief family therapy.

ERICKSON'S GOAL DIRECTEDNESS

Contrary to much therapeutic thinking, Erickson does not appear to think that an individual's symptom or complaint can usually be treated with the same approach used with other individuals who have the same symptom. His approach to human problems seems organized and governed by the different premises.

Haley (37) organized some of Erickson's cases along a continuum of the family life cycle. In this approach, problems are seen to develop as blocks to move from one life stage to the next, for example, from single adult to married adult. Haley's approach helps to illuminate one crucial aspect of Erickson's work; the therapeutic procedures are all designed with a specific goal in mind. In Haley's framework, that goal was described as moving to the next stage of the cycle.

Erickson's goal may or may not be explicit and may or may not be shared with his patient on a "conscious level." Most importantly, these goals do not seem to be exclusively symptom removal. When getting rid of a symptom is part of Erickson's design, as it usually is, this somehow seems secondary to the outcomes he reports. For instance, a woman came to Erickson with a stomach ulcer, and he helped her to stop unwanted visits from her in-laws (a truly systemic intervention). Once that "sign," or subgoal, was accomplished, the ulcer was gone as a by-product of the woman's change in her relationship with her in-laws (37).

Upon examining the cases Haley placed in each phase of the family life cycle, certain consistencies of Erickson's designs stand out. One of these constants is that Erickson's approach is determined more by the situation or context in which the person finds himself than it is by the nature of the symptom or the person's phase in the cycle. That is, the same therapeutic intervention patterns reappear with cases in various phases of the family life cycle and with various symptoms.

Although Erickson did not identify the procedures as having the same design, this metapattern can be abstracted from his particular approach to six different cases described in the literature. The symptoms cover a wide range, the problems all appear unique, and the methods Erickson used (or the metapattern described through the use of balance theory) are with people at various stages of the family life cycle: a 16-year-old thumb sucker (35, p. 428), two cases of "hysterical paralysis" (35, p. 390), an adolescent with a "big tooth" (35, p. 414), a woman with a stomach ulcer (37, p. 153), and a 21-year-old woman with a gap between her front teeth (35, p. 414).

Several features of Erickson's method in these cases deserve particular attention if we are to understand this approach, and the brief family therapy approach. In each of these cases Erickson can be described as determining a "primary goal" (say, G) for his approach, which is based on what the person offers him. In the articles, this goal is sometimes implied rather than stated. In each case this primary goal can be described in very specific terms, and it seems so constructed that the goal is within the person's world view. In systemic fashion, this primary goal is usually "interactional" in nature, not the elimination of the complaint itself. Most frequently, the complaint can be described as going away "spontaneously" through some change in the person's interactional behavior.

When establishing a primary goal, it is as though Erickson asks himself: "What can happen in this person's life so that the symptom can unobtrusively disappear?" Then, Erickson can be seen to take a step-by-step approach to reaching the goal (G) established by his answer to the above question. In Haley's framework, the question relates to a move to the next phase of the family life cycle. In the brief family therapy model, this question relates to the establishment of goals and signs.

For the woman with a stomach ulcer whom Erickson treated, the situation with her in-laws' unwanted visits changed, and then the complaint disappeared. The primary goal can be seen as the elimination of the ulcer, which was unobtrusively accomplished by the woman's changing her relationship with her in-laws.

For Erickson,

> a proper therapeutic goal is one that aids the patient to function as adequately and constructively as possible under those internal and external handicaps that constitute part of his life situation and needs. Consequently, the therapeutic task becomes a problem of intentionally utilizing neurotic symptomatology to meet the unique needs of the patient. Such utilization must . . . provide adequately for constructive adjustments aided rather than handicapped by the continuance of neuroticisms. (35, p. 390)

Each "neurotic symptom" or complaint (using this mapping technique, labeled "x") is seen to be related to the specific, primary goal (G) in at least one way: the complaint (x) can be described as somehow preventing the person from reaching that goal. At this point, we might imagine Erickson asking himself: "How can this complaint be transformed into something useful toward accomplishing the goal?"

In this step, Erickson seems interested in the manner in which "the limitations of one's usual conscious sets and belief systems are temporarily altered so that one can be receptive to an experience of other patterns of association and modes of mental functioning" (28, p. 20). His procedures, with or without the formal use of trance, promote this receptivity. His methods in this step are the "Erickson fingerprint," which allows Haley and us to know an Erickson procedure when we see one. Simply, this fingerprint involves transforming through reframing at least some aspect of the complaint from an involuntary, painful part of life into a deliberate, more useful part of life. This reframing changes the entire meaning of the person's situation, and a behavior change will follow.

For instance, a young woman had a gap between her front teeth, which she saw as repulsive and disfiguring enough to consider suicide. Rather than send her to a dentist, or try to talk her out of her suicidal thoughts, or reassure her of the minor nature of the space, Erickson taught her that the gap was uniquely useful as a tool for squirting water. When she came to therapy she was using this gap to see herself as disfigured: It was clearly beyond her control and useless. Erickson's technique started with teaching her to use the space voluntarily in a different manner.

This step in Erickson's procedure can be described as akin to a "symptom prescription" (62). In general, most complaints or symptoms can be seen as "beyond control and involuntary." A symptom prescription asks the person to perform voluntarily the symptomatic behavior (concentrating on the space between her teeth) in hopes of eliminating or at least gaining some control over the complaint. Erickson taught the young woman to use the gap voluntarily in a different manner as a step in transforming the whole situation. The goal of this step, unlike the goal of a symptom prescription, is *not* the elimination of the complaint. Rather, it is just a start in the reframing-transforming process.

This transformation is completed in the next step, which is usually a task that is instrumental in reaching the primary goal, or allows the primary goal to happen, or stops preventing the achievement of the goal. This task, or series of tasks, is built on the reframed complaint (say, x') and its new usefulness. The young lady's squirting ability was next used for a practical joke (say, G'): squirting water at a young man she had been avoiding. Here Erickson uses her ability (squirting water) as a basis for a task (the practical joke) that is dependent on the gap itself. This elicited new interactional behavior that subsequently led to the young woman's reaching her goal of marriage and children.

Through the reframing process the specific, primary goal is reached. The young woman was no longer avoiding young men who were interested in her, and she was (using Haley's frame) ready to move into the next phase of the family life cycle. The practical joke that used her gap was constructive and beneficial to her. The young woman and the young man (the victim of the joke) eventually got married. Therefore, she could no longer view the gap as repulsive and disfiguring since the gap itself helped her to reach her goal of marriage to the young man. As in other cases, Erickson's methods provided the young woman with the opportunity to reach her goal "spontaneously."

Making a Map

This approach of Erickson's can be described through the use of a balance theoretical map. (This is part of our descriptive tool, not Erickson's.) When this model was first constructed (21), the client or patient was still seen as "out there," separated from the therapist in some manner, although the therapist's relationship to the whole situation was held to be a constant (positive). The original model will be presented, first, and then it will be expanded to the eco-system.

Making a map of Erickson's procedure starts with the three elements seen from the observer's point of view—(1) the patient (say, p), (2) the primary goal (say, G), and (3) the involuntary symptom or complaint (say, x)—and (4) the *relationships* among these three elements, as illustrated in Figure 6.2.

This starting situation is mapped as a balanced state (two relations de-scribed as negative, one described as positive). The Erickson fingerprint can then be mapped as the start of the reframing process that redefines the com-plaint (x) into something more useful (say, x′). From this point, the maps can describe the goal achievement process through a subgoal (usually a task, say, G′) that used the reframed complaint (x′). The task (G′) is then mapped in rela-tion to the goal (G), shown in Figure 6.3.

It is important to realize that Erickson does not accept the person's reality in which the complaint is uncontrolled and useless (x). Instead, he accepts the complaint as part of the person's "old reality," which can be transformed so that the complaint becomes useful or even necessary for the therapeutic outcome. In using this procedure the reframed complaint (x′) is related to reaching the primary goal (G). Furthermore, he does not accept the person's goal at face value because it often is too wide in scope. Rather, he "focuses down" on a specific goal: some aspect of the person's goal that can be connected with the reframed complaint.

A description of the "gap problem" (above) can be constructed in the fol-lowing way: First, the relationship between the young woman (p) and her goal (G) can be described as positive (+) since the goal (marriage and children) is something she values. Second, the relationship between the young woman (p) and the space between her teeth (x) can be described as negative (−) since she views the gap as disfiguring enough to prompt thoughts of suicide. Third, the relationship between the gap (x) and her goal (G) can be described as negative (−) since she views the gap as preventing her from reaching her goal. In her view, desirable young men were repulsed by the gap. This configuration is la-

Figure 6.2.

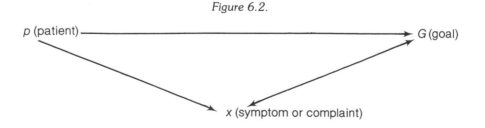

p (patient) ──────────────────────────────→ G (goal)

x (symptom or complaint)

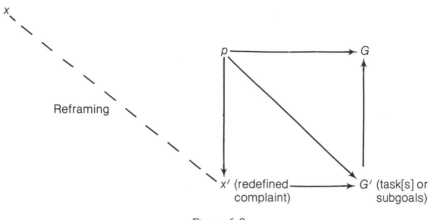

Figure 6.3.

beled a "balanced state" since two negative relations and one positive relation are described (see Figure 6.4).

The Therapy Procedure. By reframing the situation, Erickson is able to start transforming the gap into something valuable, at least for squirting water (*x'*). Then, by using that valuable asset (*x'*) to play a practical joke (*G'*), he is able to help the young woman to create a new set of relationships in which the gap can eventually come to be seen as something of value. The practical joke (*G'*) is then directly related to reaching the goal (*G*). The woman and the victim of the joke developed a relationship that eventually included marriage. When the rest of the map is positive, it is no longer viable for the young woman to maintain a negative view of the gap: It helped her reach her goal.

Figure 6.4. A balanced state.

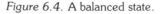

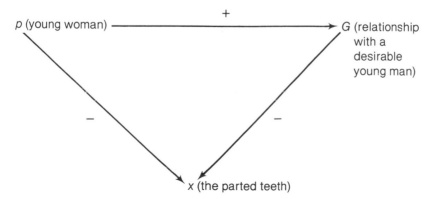

The section of the map after the reframing is described as imbalanced, which in Heider's theory means that a tendency toward balance will develop. The complaint itself has been instrumental in achieving the goal, and therefore, the relationship between the young woman and the gap will switch to positive. Described in this way, Erickson's approach can be seen to create imbalance in the original situation, which builds enough tension in the person's situation to prompt a "spontaneous" change in the relationships among the person and the complaint and the goal (see Figure 6.5).

Each of the six cases mentioned above can be described in the same fashion. Of course, Erickson's own explanations are included in the original papers, and the explanation here is not meant to conform to his. The use of balance theory as discussed here has allowed the analysis of Erickson's work to be done in such a way that it is possible to expand his principles for use in other situations.

EXTENDING THE MAP

Once the team concept developed after breaking through the mirror, this map needed to be expanded to include the whole ecosystem. It quickly became apparent that this expanded tool could serve as a "goal-directed map" for the therapy situation using the procedures and format of BFTC. Although all families and their contexts are quite different and the BFTC approach is built upon this uniqueness, the goal-directed principles of brief family therapy can be understood through the use of this mapping technique.

To extend the map through the glass, it is necessary to include the team-

Figure 6.5.

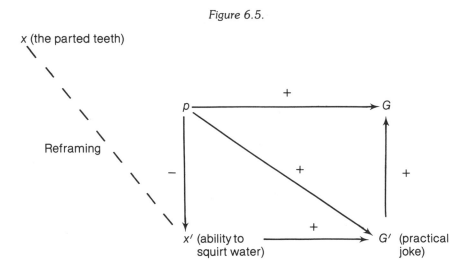

conductor unit (say, *T*) in the description. From behind the mirror and in the therapy room the team is acting to accept the family (say, *P*) and its total situation fully, including the complaint pattern (*x*). This task is accomplished by the conductor's noncritical attitude and by the compliment and clue that are based on a "positive" version of the family's situation (i.e., from a different angle).

When building the expanded map, the elements of the configuration (from a metaposition or an outside observer's position), shown in Figure 6.6, include: (*1*) the family (*p*), (*2*) the complaint pattern (*x*), (*3*) the primary goal (*G*), (*4*) the team (*T*), and (*5*) the *relationships* among these elements.

By including the team in this fashion, the therapy situation from the start can be described as placing the family (*p*) *and* its relationship to its complaint pattern (*x*) in an imbalanced situation.* On the expanded map there are two significant, additional positive relationships: (*1*) between the team (*T*) and the family (*p*) via the noncritical attitude and the compliment-clue and (*2*) between the team (*T*) and the complaint pattern (*x*) via the acceptance of the problem as normal under the circumstances and the lack of a directive calling for change.

In each case the team attempts to determine a primary goal (*G*) based on what the family has offered. This primary goal is not the elimination of the complaint pattern (*x*), but rather what it is that will happen when the complaint is no longer troubling the family. As noted before, a goal needs to be constructed as the start of something, not as the end of something. Following Erickson's example, the team will help the family *focus* on a specific goal because the family's stated goal may be too wide in scope. The question the team asks itself is: "What can happen in this family's situation so that the complaint can unobtrusively disappear?" The answer helps to define the goal.

Each complaint and the interaction pattern that surrounds the complaint (*x*) is described as related to a primary goal (*G*) in some way. The complaint pattern (*x*) is somehow preventing the family (*p*) from achieving the goal. The team members ask this question: "How can this pattern be reframed into something (*x'*) that will start a process that allows the family to achieve the goal?"

The process from the initial reframing (leading to *x'*) to the development of the signs (*G'*) can involve a series of messages from the team aimed at the sub-

---

*Although the entire map (Figure 6.6) can be described as balanced (an even number of negative signs), the team-family-complaint subsystem or area of the map is imbalanced (only one negative sign attributed). The therapy procedure can be seen to operate on this limited area of the map. Every conceptual scheme must take a chunk of the wider ecosystem for methodological purposes, otherwise the data supply becomes immense.

This particular chunking seems heuristically useful for conceptualizing therapeutic procedures. As a safeguard, compliments and clues are phrased without mention of goals, and only this section of the map obtains in the first session.

The reframing process, begun by the compliment and clue at the end of the first session, is an attempt to "create a new reality" and therefore a new map (Figure 6.7), which is imbalanced (line *p* to *x'*) enough to have tendencies to seek balance and thus goal achievement.

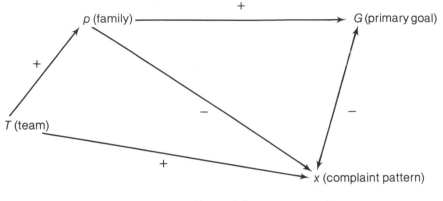

Figure 6.6.

goals. This can be some unobtrusive event that allows or promotes the achieve-ment of the goal (G), or it can be the specifically named signs (G') (see Figure 6.7).

Guidelines

From this description of Erickson's procedure and its adaptation to brief family therapy, guidelines have been developed to assist therapist's efforts to be goal directed.

1. The negatively evaluated complaint pattern (x) is important and pain-ful to the family (p).
2. The family (p) describes the complaint pattern (x) as beyond its control.
3. The primary goal (G) must be acceptable within the family's world view. This goal can be subject to negotiation, can sometimes be im-plied, or can be hypothesized by the team (T).
4. The family must accept of the specific, primary goal, stated or implied. The goal (G) must be positively evaluted by the family.
5. The team (T) must noncritically accept the family (p) and its world view. This acceptance must include the complaint pattern (x).
6. The team (T) shifts the definition of the involuntary complaint pattern (x) by reframing toward some version of this pattern (x') that is more useful and/or more voluntary.
7. The team either develops or prompts the development of a new use for this reframed, more useful aspect of the complaint pattern (x'). The more useful aspect is then instrumental in achieving the signs of pro-gress or the subgoals (G').

8. The subgoals (G') must either be instrumental in achieving the primary goal (G) or allow the achieving of the goal.
9. Evaluation of the voluntary aspect (x') is changed in a positive direction. The family has either gained control of the complaint pattern or the complaint pattern has been eliminated.

A CASE EXAMPLE

Session 1

During the first two sessions, Mr. and Mrs. Quill complained about their girls' behavior in various situations. While this description was going on, Mary (aged 8) and Debbie (aged 6) were running around the therapy room exploring the surface of the mirror with their faces and hands and bickering with each other. At very infrequent invervals either mother or father would ask the girls to stop doing something, but this was either ignored or, if the girls responded, it was only momentary. Debbie climbed all over her father while he was talking; he stoically maintained his calm as he continued to describe their situation. Periodically he would interrupt his descriptions to ask Debbie to stop climbing on him, but to no avail. At no time during the first session was either parent effective in stopping the girls' behavior for more than a moment or two.

Figure 6.7.

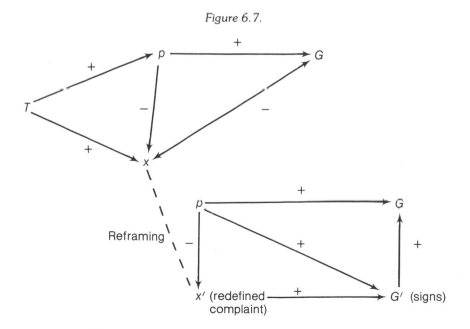

The team complimented the parents on their task-centered focus and the girls on their inquisitiveness and their ability to explore on their own. Once they showed their acceptance of the compliments, the parents were asked to "think about what you are sure that you do *not* want to change about the parent-child relationships (the parents' terms) in your family."

Sometimes this task can have interesting results. It is very difficult to think about what you do *not* want to change without thinking about what you *do* want to change. Since the Quill family's complaints were expressed in global terms (get the girls to behave better), the team will attempt to help them get more specific. If Mr. and Mrs. Quill can respond to this task by describing what they do not want to change (a straightforward response report), then the team will have more and better information about the family's frame and its manner of cooperating. An opposite response report might help Mr. and Mrs. Quill give the team a more focused version of their complaints, thus giving the team information about their manner of cooperating. Furthermore, there is an implication in this clue that neither the girls, nor their parents, nor the interaction between parents and girls is totally bad in the eyes of the team.

The Quill family's situation in the first session can be mapped, using the balance theoretical maps, as follows: The family's (p) goal (G) was stated as "getting the girls to behave better." The complaint pattern (x) centered around the girls' misbehavior and the parents' attempts to deal with this behavior, which was shown to be ineffective. The team showed its acceptance of the Quill family's situation by being noncritical throughout the session and by the compliment. Further, the team showed its acceptance of some aspects of the complaint pattern by focusing on the "positive" side of the observed interaction patterns. The clue started the reframing by implying there was something "good" about the very thing about which the parents were complaining—the parent-child relationships (Figure 6.8).

Session 2

At the start of the second session Debbie arranged the seating. This involved mother's moving from one chair to another despite her protests and father's picking up a chair and moving it to a new location. The conductor carefully did not interfere; he just observed. Subsequently, mother and Mary began a discussion about a hassle that occurred the previous day. Debbie was sitting between them and interrupted the conversation frequently. The conductor called Debbie over to him and asked Mary to switch chairs. Throughout the next 30 minutes, Mr. Quill attempted to keep the girls in this new formation. Mrs. Quill did not join in this attempt.

Later, Mrs. Quill said that she did not consider the seating important

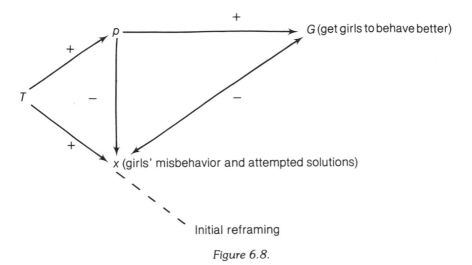

Figure 6.8.

enough, and she thought that if she were to get involved, then she would have gotten angry and would have yelled at the girls. She did not want to do this. When the girls finally sat still in Debbie's chair and became quiet, Mrs. Quill suggested that father should accept this as a resolution, which he did reluctantly. (This activity during the session confirmed for the team that the parents' description of the complaint pattern fit the sequences the team observed.)

Concurrently, the conductor attempted to check out the Quill's response to the task. Mrs. Quill's response centered around not wanting Mary to "change into a small adult or an automoton." When the girls were in a good mood, she found them enjoyable. She went on to complain that these good moods were only in anticipation of, or in reaction to, a special happening. Mr. Quill complained that these "good moods" were often "too high"; the girls would run around the house yelling and screaming. He wanted to start from "ground zero and change everything." (Neither of them reported any role he or she might have had in these situations. They focused entirely on the girls' behavior, missing the clue's emphasis on the interaction between parents and children. Therefore, the team described their response report as "modified.")

The team complimented Mr. and Mrs. Quill on having found ways to teach their children to think independently and on their persistance on this task in the face of any difficulties this learning might accidentally produce. A clue was designed to get further details about the interaction patterns at home and to help Mr. and Mrs. Quill focus a bit. They were instructed to alternate roles for one hour during the evening on five of the next seven days. The other days they were told to behave as usual. During this hour, one parent was to be in charge of any and all problems, while the other parent was to pretend he or she was not there. The observing parent was to take note of any urges to interfere and any actual times he or she did interfere.

This is an easily modifiable task. Anything the parents might observe and describe about their parts in the sequence would be helpful to the team, and the observations were the team's objective. The team had hopes that this task would produce some information about what the parents actually did. Furthermore, the task attempted to limit Mrs. Quill's interference when Mr. Quill was dealing with the girls.

Session 3

This session was scheduled for the parents only, and they reported that on two evenings during the interval they were able to perform the assignment. As demonstrated during the second session, they reported that Mr. Quill was unable to be effective with Mary. On one occasion Mrs. Quill had to help out because Mary refused to deal with her father. This was a shock to both of them. Again their observations centered around the girls' behavior. Neither Mr. nor Mrs. Quill was able to think of anything he or she could do to change his or her situation; and both felt hopeless.

The Quills' puzzle was framed around the discipline of the girls, mainly Mary. Whatever they tried failed to be effective. They very seldom resorted to spanking because they did not want the girls to be angry. The team's job is to reframe this puzzle in such a way that it becomes solvable. The parents continued to look at the girls' behavior and did not see the other end of the circle—their own behavior. The parents saw only the end of the sequence where they attempted to discipline the girls. On the other hand, the team punctuated the "start" of the sequence as when the parents made a request for the girls to behave. If, for instance, the parents could "start" the sequence in a different way, a change of key, then they might get some changes in the girls' behavior. The team decided to continue reframing the situation into one in which the parents needed to get the girls' attention at the very start of the sequence rather than to try to make the parents' discipline more effective. The latter would not be a difference that made a difference but "more of the same." Since Mr. and Mrs. Quill's way of cooperating as shown to the team was to modify the direct tasks, the team decided that the clue should be highly modifiable.

After the report on the response to the previous clue and some general talk about their efforts to help the girls behave, mother explained her "soft approach." She expressed the hope that if she continued doing what she was already doing, it would eventually work. Therefore (from the recording):

> MRS. QUILL: They won't blame us later for being mean.
> CONDUCTOR: Maybe you don't have to be mean. Why would you have to be mean?

MRS. QUILL: They'll be angry if we're denying them something they want to do.

CONDUCTOR: Oh, yeah. I'm not sure you have to be mean. Let me tell you about one family. They decided they were going to. . . . Let's see, how old was that kid? About so high; five or six. In that range. Well, this kid had, not only did he have mother and father convinced that he was a "holy terror" and could terrorize them into whatever he wanted them to do, but he had the upstairs neighbors and the neighbors across the street convinced also. One day, mother decided to go out and buy a squirt gun. Interestingly enough, the same day father did too.

They didn't want to beat up on the kid's bottom, so they decided something had to happen. They didn't tell each other they were going to buy squirt guns. Mother told the kid to do something. The kid said "no," and she walked away and got her squirt gun. Then she told the kid to do it again, then zapped him with the squirt gun and walked away. This time he went and did it. Funny thing: When father came home, he too had a squirt gun. He told the kid to stop doing something. When the kid said "no" father didn't even wait. He emptied the gun on the kid. And then told him that was just the start of it. The kid stopped.

They kept the squirt guns around for whenever they were determined they wanted the kid's attention, they would zap him with the squirt gun first, before saying anything.

MRS. QUILL: Did they zap him over everything? Like finishing the milk?

CONDUCTOR: I don't know where they drew the line.

Then another family. Their main complaint was about two little kids. I guess they were six and nine. These kids would get into hassles between themselves and into this stomping stuff. Typically, mother would go in there and yell at the kids to "Shut up!" Well, she got awfully tired of that. It didn't work too well, as you know.

So, one day she decided that she was trying to treat these kids like they were much older than they really were, and that they did not really understand her when she told them to stop fighting. She said to herself, "My goodness, there must be a way I can get down on their level," but she couldn't think of anything. So, she wandered off into the kitchen and there was this big three-gallon pot. And, she says, "Ah ha!" So, the next time these kids got into a big noisy hassle, she grabbed the pot and a wooden spoon. She snuck up to where the kids were fighting, and she banged on the pot until they shut up. She said, "Thank you," and went back into the kitchen. A couple of days of that, and at least the kids' fights were a lot quieter and didn't bother her so much. I don't know when the kids stopped fighting.

MR. QUILL: We did something once when the kids were arguing. We started to argue too. So, they started sitting there, staring at us, wondering what was going on. I guess we never did that again, though it did work.

On their way out of the office, Mrs. Quill asked her husband where they might get squirt guns. Throughout this story telling, both were obviously amused and intrigued by the clues being presented. Their acceptance was demonstrated by smiles and nods and further confirmed by Mr. Quill's story.

At no time during the session were they told to use either of these "gimmicks" to get the girls' attention, and, therefore, this is a very modifiable task. The conductor was just telling them stories about how somewhat similar families had solved their somewhat similar problems: how to get their kids' attention without being mean. These stories were isomorphic with the family's situation, and the different angle is presented by the methods the other families used to solve the problem. If Mr. and Mrs. Quill were to decide to use either or both gimmicks, the choice was theirs to make. Either of these gimmicks might significantly affect the complaint patterns and the parents' perception of the situation. Of course, if they did use the gimmicks, this would be a sign to the team that the intervention was isomorphic and in line with the family's demonstrated manner of cooperating. That is, the different angle of the intervention would provide the Quills with an idea that led to a different behavior, which then can be seen to promote further changes in the interaction with the children.

Follow-Up

Mr. and Mrs. Quill did buy the squirt guns on their way home. They lost little time before trying out that trick to get the girls' attention. It was successful (see Figure 6.9). As is frequently the case, Mr. and Mrs. Quill treated the squirt gun story as though it had been a direct task. That is, they modified the indirect suggestions into direct suggestions. The conductor denied that he gave them a direct task and expressed surprise that they took the stories so seriously. He only told them those stories to let them know they were not alone in the world and to let them know that other people had found surprising ways to cope. Two subsequent sessions in the next two months confirmed that Mr. and Mrs. Quill had initiated a new pattern. They were now able to get the girls' attention in various ways, and they did not have to resort to anything "mean" in the way of discipline. Both the parents and the school reported better behavior.

Mrs. Quill had also been "inspired" by the pot-banging gimmick, but this was not within her range of behavior. As she said, "I could never do that." Instead, she bought a referree's whistle to use in the same manner (another way of modifying the task).

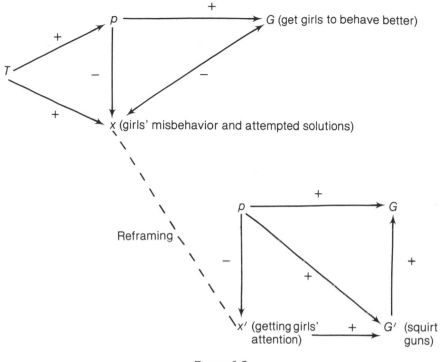

Figure 6.9.

Comment. By reframing the complaint as a problem of gaining the girls attention (x') the team was at least able to not be critical of the parents' methods. The problem of gaining the girls' attention (x') was able to be dealt with through the squirt gun gimmick and the whistle (G') and, therefore, a new pattern was established that allowed the family to reach its goal (G) of getting the girls to behave better.

The type of indirect task used as a clue in this case is similar to the indirect suggestions Erickson often used in hypnotherapy, ones that utilize "a patient's own associative structure and mental skills in ways that are outside his usual range of conscious ego control to effect therapeutic goals" (28, p. 311). Furthermore, Erickson's idea of trance suggests "that fixing and focusing attention by such conversation does put the listener into trance without the need for any other formal process of induction" (28, p. 311).

An indirect clue needs to be so constructed that the "story" relates to the family's patterns in an isomorphic manner but from that different angle. That is, the patterns in the "story's family" should be similar in detail to the patterns the family is complaining about. Debbie and Mary could "terrorize" Mr. and Mrs.

Quill into whatever the girls wanted, just like the kid in the story. Similarly, the parents in the story did not want to beat the kid's bottom, just like the Quill's who did not want to do anything mean. Mary and Debbie got into frequent hassles—yelled and screamed at each other and stomped off when upset. And Mrs. Quill would yell at them to "shut up." All of these were made part of the story.

The different angle is provided by the unique solutions the "story families" found. Therefore, when the family pattern erupts in the Quill household, Mr. and Mrs. Quill can be stimulated by this news of a difference. That is, they are likely "automatically" to associate their patterns with the clues hidden in the stories, which might prompt them either to perceive the situation differently or to do something differently. In this way the indirect clue is similar to a posthypnotic suggestion that Erickson usually associated with everyday events in a seemingly casual manner. This connection between pattern and clue increases the likelihood that the person will perform the suggested act. If there was little or no connection, the odds would probably be against having any person perform a posthypnotic suggestion, and, therefore, the odds would likely be against any family performing a suggested task.

The Jay Family

Chapters 7 and 8 are devoted to a session-by-session study of the therapy processes with two families. In both chapters, the sessions are broken down into the sections of the format used at BFTC. This method will help to clarify the relationship between what the conductor does and what the team behind the mirror does while in interaction with the family.

All of the quotations in Chapter 7 and 8 are from videotapes made of each session with the families' full knowledge and consent. Of course, the families are disguised to prevent recognition, while the essential details are retained. Only minor changes have been made in the script to clarify who is speaking and to whom.

In this chapter, which is about the therapy with the Jay family, there are two conductors in the room with the family: James F. Derks and Byron McBride.* This is an exception to BFTC's usual practice of having only one conductor in the room. There are two reasons for this exception: (1) Mrs. Jay had seen McBride privately in individual therapy four years earlier, and (2) McBride was not a member of the BFTC staff. He anticipated that this would be a rough case and, therefore, brought the family to BFTC with him.

A CASE STUDY

After an interval of four years, Mrs. Jay returned for therapy because she was once again having somatic complaints, and she was again disturbed by the difficulty one of her children was having in leaving home. McBride saw this as a repeat of the old pattern, and, therefore, he decided on a different approach.

Prior to the first session, Derks and the rest of the team† did not know who was coming in for the session. The team only knew about the somatic complaints and the difficulty the daughter was having in leaving home at age 21. As

---

*A psychologist in private practice in Milwaukee.
†Behind the mirror were de Shazer and Diane Scharp and Jo Ellyn Schultz, both of whom were in training at BFTC.

a temporary map, the team hypothesized that the youngest daughter might be described as sacrificing herself to protect her parents from having to be alone without any of the children at home. Therefore, perhaps she could be described as attempting to keep her parents' marriage together. On the other hand, perhaps mother and father were protecting their daughter from having to face the cold cruel world alone. (It is important to remember that maps are only useful tools. Neither accuracy nor truth are to be inferred. "Motivations," such as the ones this map suggests, are always to be read "as if." That is, the daughter's behavior might be understood "as if" she were acting to protect the marriage, etc.)

Prelude to Session 1

When the family arrived, Derks introduced them to BFTC's operation: the one-way mirror, the video equipment, and the presence of a team behind the mirror. Mr. Jay was the supervisor in a plant and had held that job for many years. He enjoyed his line of work. He seemed to be a pleasant man with a well-developed sense of humor that he used to advantage as a member of a theater group. Mrs. Jay looked worn and hassled. She worked part-time as a house parent with disturbed adolescents. Joan (aged 25) was a college senior who was optimistic about her future. She was slightly overweight and quite cheerful in demeanor. Joan worked part-time with young children. She lived down the block from her parents' home. Jane (aged 21) was employed part-time as an assistant manager in a chain store, a job she disliked. During the early part of the session she was rather quiet. Mike Jr. (aged 22) was currently a psychiatric inpatient. The team learned that he was married and managed the apartment house across the street from the Jay family home.

Data Collecting

Derks signaled the shift from the prelude by asking the Jays: "Well, what brings you here?" while he faced McBride. Mrs. Jay responded, "Mainly me." When Mrs. Jay was taking their deaf and blind dog (that they had had for 13 years) out for a walk, he was killed by a car.

> MRS. JAY: I should have had him on a chain, but I didn't. I yelled, "Stay," but he didn't hear me.

The dog died on the way to the vet. Mrs. Jay started to hyperventilate and felt very guilty about the dog's death. Mr. Jay took her to a hospital where she received treatment. He had expected them to keep her overnight, but they surprised him when she was released immediately.

MR. JAY: We worry a lot about Martha. She's hypertensive.

The girls and Mr. Jay quickly jumped to mother's defense. She should not feel guilty about the dog's death since it was not unusual to walk the dog without a chain, and it was because of the dog's deafness and blindness that he did not see or hear the car.

Although Martha could be as "cool as a cucumber about a lot of things," she developed psychosomatic symptoms, she said, about the things that really upset her. After the dog's death she continued to feel a tightness in her chest and was gasping for air when she called McBride. Mr. Jay wanted to see Martha through all this because her "coping mechanisms were not too strong."

Prior to the dog's death, Junior had started acting crazy. During a cold spell, he walked barefoot the eight miles to his grandmother's home. He was described as "delusional," and the family sought professional help. His wife was described as "not too bright." Mrs. Jay had known her daughter-in-law for years as a member of the girl scout troop. However, they clearly stated that Junior and his problems were not what had brought them to therapy: The problem was Mrs. Jay.

It seemed that it was difficult for the Jay children to leave home. Joan lived down the block and Junior across the street. At the same time Jane started to take steps toward leaving home, Junior started to "act crazy," while mother became depressed and had somatic symptoms exacerbated by the death of dog. Dad stoically supported mother through all these events.

At this point, it seemed that the family was showing a willingness to support mother through these "troublesome times" and that the family could be described as "allowing her to sacrifice herself by carrying the major share of the pain" by feeling depressed and guilty while having somatic complaints. Mr. Jay would stand behind her and absolve her from blame.

The Jay family situation can best be described through looking at the dog's death incident. The dog's death is not seen as mother's fault; since the dog was deaf, he could not be expected to hear her call, "Stay." She had done her best. The two girls joined father in absolving mother from this responsibility, pointing out that none of them used a chain when walking the dog. Therefore, mother could be "guilty" without being guilty in the eyes of the rest of the family. Since, in this description, mother's reality is being denied by the family, perhaps she could feel depressed and have somatic complaints: ways of suffering that did not need the family's confirmation.

This kind of disqualification has often been described as a "trademark" of families with a "high level of disturbance." The "defense against blame" by a transfer similar to the dog incident was described by Haley (33) as part of his model of the schizophrenic family, which might reasonably be extended to other families with a "high degree of disturbance."

Derks asked Joan how leaving home had been for her. Mrs. Jay responded that it happened after a "tiff." Joan's version was different: It was a big fight, not a tiff. Mr. Jay remembered neither. At that time, Joan had not been doing well in school, and she went to live with an uncle for nine months during which time none of her immediate family spoke to her.

> MRS. JAY: So, it was not your idea to leave.
> MRS. JAY: And, we didn't throw you out.

Everybody agreed. (Another defense against blame, a redundant sequence.) Joan subsequently returned home for a brief period before moving to the apartment down the block. At this point, Mr. Jay introduced his "theme song."

> MR. JAY: I've always held that when a child reaches a certain age, they
>   should go out on their own. For their own good, not just for Mom and
>   Dad's rest—which they have coming. One of these days, Jane will be
>   asked to leave. This will be harder on mother, harder than on father.
> JANE: I'll probably move out one of these days.
> JOAN: But there's a double message here. You want Jane to move out
>   sometime, but you just built a new bed for her which is permanent. A
>   very nice bed which can't be moved.
> JANE: It makes a better house.
> JOAN: That's what it is suppose to mean.
> JANE: I didn't take it to mean I've gotta stay there.

There were denials of any intention other than fixing up the house. The built-in bed was only an improvement in case they decided to sell the house.

The team was struck by the repeat of the responsibility theme. Father could *say* that children should move out on their own, but not *do* anything about that notion. In fact, he could actively undermine the whole idea by making the child's bed a permanent part of the house "just as an improvement." Mother then could actively fear what might happen if Jane did move out. In this way, father can be described as if he is protecting mother from Jane's moving out, while he also protected Jane from leaving. Jane's staying could also be described as though she were protecting mother and father by not leaving. Mother showed that she felt the "brunt of it all," which can be described as though she is protecting father from something while helping to keep Jane at home and protecting her from attempting to live on her own and failing. Joan seemed detached enough from this to comment upon all this, but her comments were rejected or disqualified by mother, father, and Jane.

Their worries were certainly real enough. Jane had periodically threatened suicide and had made several attempts that were all described as responses to breaking up with various boy friends. And when mother worries about this, she gets somatic symptoms.

> MR. JAY: As I said, leaving is harder on mother than it is on father. We all love Jane, and don't want to see anything happen. But there comes a time when a child should leave home.

Goals. All four agreed that the main goal of therapy was to help mother feel less depressed. When Derks asked how they would know Mrs. Jay was less depressed, the family members came up with various signs. If Martha were not depressed, then (1) she would take more interest in things and (2) she would take better care of the house. Jane thought (3) she would know for sure when mother and father did some traveling or went on a canoe trip. Joan thought (4) she would know for sure when she came over and there was some pleasant conversation rather than talk about problems. She also thought a good sign would be (5) a decrease in mother's blood pressure. Mr. Jay agreed with these, and he added that a good sign would be (6) when they both felt enough energy to lose some weight. Mrs. Jay thought she would know for sure she was less depressed when (7) she started working more hours or actually did go back to school.

Right before the break, Mrs. Jay declared that she felt like she was "sitting on a balloon waiting for it to break" or "like she was waiting for the next bomb to fall."

Consulting Break

The team was surprised that Jane's leaving was not mentioned as either a sign or a goal. Also surprising was that none of the goals involved Junior. The entire focus was around Mrs. Jay.

The signs and goal suggested that the Jays' way of cooperating might well include this focus on mother's depression and somatic complaints. Whatever the suprasystem pattern might become, the initial focus should be on these complaints and on the supporting behavior of the others in order to be isomorphic. The intervention needs to include something about helping mother to cope, and it should not include anything suggesting a change in the supportive stance.

The family's goal was clear: Help mother to be less depressed. The family members had developed seven signs that would indicate to them that mother was starting to be nondepressed. The team's intervention should help the family take a small step in that direction.

Since there was also a difficulty around leaving home, the team inferred that the family had strong values around "staying together." The team also noted that things "sort of happened" to the Jays and that the whole family never considered anybody to be responsible for these events.

The team decided that the compliment should be built on the idea of "keeping the family together" and that the clue should develop mother's balloon metaphor, which would include the alternate ways a balloon can lose air—slow or quick. Further, the team decided not to be specific about what might happen once the balloon lost air. In this way a situation is created in which an empty balloon might be a desired outcome. It was for this reason that the team chose the balloon rather than the bomb metaphor. A bomb is destructive, and a flat balloon is not. Therefore, should anybody do anything to "burst the balloon," the team might have the option of reframing that in a beneficial way, whereas a bomb might be difficult to so relabel.

Message Giving

MR. JAY: What did they tell you?

MRS. JAY: No hope, huh? (*The whole family laughed.*)

McBRIDE: We were all impressed with the efforts you've all made to keep this family together through all these crises. A lot of families would just fall apart under all this pressure. It's a pretty overwhelming bunch of problems that could blow many families into little pieces.

DERKS: We are all concerned about your balloon. We think it might burst soon, though Steve, behind the mirror there, says it might just develop a slow leak. What we would like you all to do is watch for signs that it's going to burst, or that a slow leak is developing.

MR. JAY: Would it be better if it was a slow leak?

DERKS: I don't know. If it's slow, it might be painful. If it's fast, it might be a shock. I would think a slow leak would be better, but Steve seemed more worried about a slow leak.

MR. JAY: We don't want you people to get into arguments over our balloon.

The Jays all agreed to watch for signs that either a slow leak or a sudden burst were starting to develop and the next appointment was set.

Behind the mirror, the team observed the family showing signs of accepting both parts of the message. The team was convinced that the intervention was at least close to the family's manner of cooperating and was roughly isomorphic

Study Efforts

After the family left, the team met to discuss the immediate responses to the messages that the family had shown. The team predicted that the Jay family would return for the next appointment and that it would report having watched Martha for signs of the balloon losing air. The team also predicted that another crisis might develop—a burst balloon.

Comment. The intervention was designed to accept the Jays' current situation. Although Mr. Jay had introduced the idea that Jane should move out, the family was seen to pull together against this notion when this was brought up—thus the compliment on the status quo.

The observation task was built on the Jays' pattern of watching and supporting mother while she carried the brunt of the problem. The team's effort to expand the metaphor through expanding the watchfulness to include a slow leak was meant to imply that things might get better, thus providing a potentially different angle from which to observe and be concerned about Martha. The team expected the Jays to follow this task in a straightforward manner.

Session 2

When the Jays arrived, it was obvious that Mrs. Jay was upset, and she appeared to be more depressed. Jane seemed to have been drinking, and she sat quietly in the corner during the first part of the session. Joan had to work and therefore did not come to the session.

MRS. JAY: We're not in a very good space. It seems that the rest of the family doesn't want family therapy. So, I guess we'll have to switch back to individual. Joan was willing to come, but she had to work. She's not really part of the problem, anyway.

DERKS: It's a good sign that she's independent enough to make that decision herself.

MR. JAY: I don't know if it will help much. I just went along for Martha's sake.

MRS. JAY: We're here about my anxieties, anyway.

So, once again, Martha is showing that she is being called upon to sacrifice, and the other members of the family will reluctantly support her.

When Derks asked about their having seen any signs of the balloon losing air, Jane reported that she had seen none until that very evening when mother seemed much more depressed. Martha and Mike had seen signs of increasing pressure and thought it was still building. They were waiting for it to burst.

One of the signs of increasing pressure developed when Mr. and Mrs. Jay learned that they were responsible for some of Junior's debts. Mr. Jay had co-signed for a loan, and the payments were behind. Both parents felt responsible for these debts and for the problems the children had.

MR. JAY: It's the maternal instinct to keep the family together. Now, I think they should go out on their own. We brought them up to be independent.

MRS. JAY: I'd like them to be on their own. I don't think we did a real good job of raising the kids to be independent.

Various attempts the children had made to be more independent had ended in some type of trouble for both parents and child. Throughout the early part of the session, Martha was crying (without visible tears) while Jane showed signs of being more and more uncomfortable. Finally, Jane blamed herself for all the problems in the family and precipitously left the session, but only after her parents had absolved her of blame.

MRS. JAY: I'm afraid of any of them getting hurt.

MR. JAY: If it was a nice transition, it would be fine with Martha.

MCBRIDE: Everybody seems to pull together when things go wrong.

MR. JAY: I'd like to get rid of them, but if we try . . . Jane threatens suicide.

DERKS: Jane keeps a pin right up to the edge of the balloon. Maybe it's easier to live with that, than to throw them out.

MCBRIDE: Like mother birds do.

MRS. JAY: I wish I could do that.

The family's response report to the rather metaphorical task was straightforward: They did observe the signs. The predicted crisis seemed to be in process. Both Mrs. Jay and Jane can be described as though continuing to sacrifice themselves to keep the family together. The drinking was bound to "cause" mother and father to remain involved with Jane because her threats of suicide were often associated with her drinking. Martha continued crying on and off during the session, and Mike held her hand at several points, a noted difference between the first and second sessions. The team was concerned that Mike would pull out of therapy, which could be described as protecting the family by continuing the pattern of letting Martha carry the brunt of the problem. Therefore, any intervention the team designs needs to be as circular as possible while continuing to describe the Jays' experience of reality.

Any intervention also needs to follow the family pattern of absolving all from any blame in order for the message to be isomorphic. The message also needed to comment on the independence theme.

Immediately before the break, Mike and Martha talked about a new house they were thinking about buying. They liked a smaller house because they would not need all the room once the children were gone.

Consulting Break

(During the break, the Jays pulled their chairs together, and Mike held Martha in his arms while she continued to cry. The team silently cheered.)

The whole team was concerned about keeping Mike in therapy. It was decided to base the intervention on a simplified map, shown in Figure 7.1, of the couple's interaction pattern. An intervention based on this map would describe Martha's depression as protecting Mike from visibly suffering, while Mike's "stiff upper lip" protects her from being overwhelmed by just how deeply he cares; information that he thinks—if she knew about—would only make her more depressed. This map needs to be extended to connect this pattern with their effort to hold the family together.

Since Martha, in the first session, and Mike, in the second, had each brought up new information after the conductors had announced the break, the team decided to have a "tag," or an additional therapeutic message, available should they bring up more new information after the intervention was delivered. Since they brought up moving and mother had used the phrase "too full nest," the tag was built on these pieces of information and the family name.

Message Giving

McBRIDE: We're all impressed with your concern for being good parents and your efforts to help them be independent and self-reliant. There's no doubt you tried.

MRS. JAY: But our track record isn't very good.

McBRIDE: But you did try. It's natural for you to feel responsible when the kids get in trouble. (To Mike) In spite of your concern that family therapy won't work, you've supported her through this.

DERKS: We realize that riding this balloon puts a lot of pressure on you [Martha] and that your efforts to hold the family together are a great sacrifice. We suspect that your depressed feelings somehow protect Mike from being overwhelmed by these troublesome times.

Further, we suspect that Mike's stiff upper lip, in spite of his upset feelings, protects you from being overwhelmed by these troublesome times.

And, these troublesome times may be just damned back luck.

MR. AND MRS. JAY: Yeah!

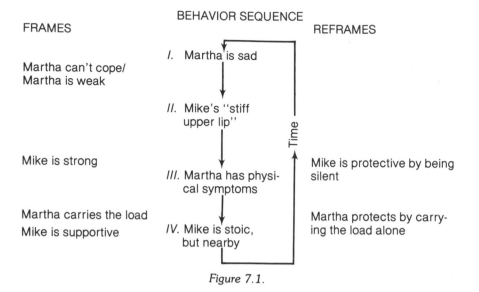

FRAMES

BEHAVIOR SEQUENCE

REFRAMES

I. Martha is sad

Martha can't cope/
Martha is weak

II. Mike's "stiff
upper lip"

Time

Mike is strong

III. Martha has physi-
cal symptoms

Mike is protective by being
silent

Martha carries the load
Mike is supportive

IV. Mike is stoic,
but nearby

Martha protects by carry-
ing the load alone

Figure 7.1.

McBride then suggested that Mike come and listen to Martha's therapy. Mike agreed, saying, "It's at least a night out." The team phoned in that Mike should also take Martha out to dinner on this "night out." Both smiled.

The Jays continued the conversation as the conductors led them out of the room. As the Jays went down the front steps, McBride gave them the "tag"; "Oh, by the way, Steve says that maybe you should move the nest." They laughed and said they would continue to think about that.

When the conductors returned from the break, Martha was still upset and tearful. While the message was being delivered, the team observed that Martha's mood brightened when the idea was introduced that Mike was protecting her. When the "damned bad luck" idea was introduced, both of them showed visible relief. They were joking on their way out of the office.

Study Effort

At this point the team felt some confidence in its description of the patterns, and the different angle of the message seemed to have shown some immediate effect. Since the Jays had responded in a straightfoward manner to the first task, the team predicted another straightforward response. The team predicted that the Jays would show some clear changes during the next session and that they would report some changes as occurring during the interval.

What specific changes might be reported were impossible to predict. The intervention seemed to be isomorphic enough and from a different angle to prompt a difference that would make a difference.

Session 3

When Mr. and Mrs. Jay came in they both appeared more cheerful and relaxed. After some social chitchat, they described the events of the previous night. At 2:00 A.M., Jane called. She was at a party in the suburbs and had no way of getting home. Mike agreed to take the 10-mile trip to pick her up. It turned out to be a pleasant drive for Martha and Mike, although Jane was not there when they arrived. Martha described it as a beautiful drive, and they had a nice conversation. The episode confirmed for both of them that Jane needed to leave the Jays' nest.

> DERKS: So it turned out like a date?
> MRS. JAY: Oh, we had one of those too!

During the week between sessions, Mike and Martha had gone bowling and out to dinner. They both enjoyed the "date," and the conversation did not include problems.

Since the episode the previous night, Mr. and Mrs. Jay had talked about Jane. Both now were angry and agreed that Jane needed to move out soon. The remainder of the session focused on how they were going to tell Jane that now was the time for her to move. Martha was convinced that Jane had to move further than two blocks away since the last time Jane lived away from home she came back and stole things; Mike had since changed all the locks. The Jays were well aware that Jane probably would cause some problems when she was told to move out, and, therefore, Mike had decided to tell her when Martha was at work. Martha objected to this plan: "Mike, don't protect me."

The team's predictions had been on target. The Jays were showing some changes, all of which were in line with the signs of progress: Martha had worked more hours; her blood pressure was down; and they had had some pleasant conversations. The response report on the previous task was rather straightforward: the date and the dinner, which is a slight modification (which the team needs to keep in mind). Martha was also showing signs of feeling less depressed, and she had reported feeling better.

The team agreed with the Jays that Jane would likely continue to do something in reaction to a "move-out message." Jane would probably raise hell, particularly if she thought they were divided on the issue: actions that could be described as though she were attempting to keep the family together.

Mike had decided that the message to Jane needed to include a deadline, and he had picked two weeks.

> MRS. JAY: When we tell her to leave, she'll give us the works. But I'll learn to cope somehow, even if she should carry through with suicide threats.
>
> MR. JAY: We did the best we could. It's out of my hands.
>
> McBRIDE: Parents are like bows. The job is done when the arrow has left the string.

Martha and Mike laughed, and the conductors took a break.

Consulting Break

The team was concerned about the possible reactions Jane might have to the "move-out message" with a deadline. Threats of suicide, of quitting her job, or of getting drunk and hurting herself thus landing in jail or a psychiatric hospital or a successful suicide were all possibilities. Martha and Mike were well aware of these possibilities, and, therefore, they did not need to be warned in the message. Martha and Mike had two immediate difficulties facing them; (1) that suicide threats would prevent them from delivering the message or (2) that once they delivered the message, they might back down and let Jane stay. Either of these would be indications that their old frame was still in place or in place again; thus, Martha would likely become depressed again, and the old pattern could repeat. The team needs to be aware of the possibility of such a recurrence and, therefore, needs to predict it or schedule it so that the family is not surprised. All of these considerations went into developing the intervention.

Comment. A this point, the team could easily get sidetracked into a new goal: helping the Jays get Jane successfully moved out. However, the girl's moving out was not one of the family's goals and was not one of the signs of progress they chose. Subsequently, the family is making the connection between the girl's moving out and Martha's difficulties. Of course, Jane's moving out might be a real strong sign of change, if the transition is different. If the Jays want the team's help in helping Jane move out, the team's efforts must be to construct this help within the context of the original goals.

Should Jane not move out (for whatever reason), the therapy could still be successful if the original signs and goal were met. Jane's move could be seen as a natural pattern (of the family life cycle) but so could her staying at home *if* her remaining did not cause Martha to be depressed or have somatic complaints and did not cause Mike to develop a stiff upper lip. If both parents and Jane define her staying home in such a way that it is not a problem and they all define Jane as an adult who chooses to stay home, then there is no need for the child to move. Historically, many unmarried adult children have remained at home *without* being defined as a child.

Message Giving

> DERKS: We were impressed by your ability, Mike, to keep your anger at Jane in check, and we think you should continue to do so, until just the right time. It's probably not wise to spread it around. Martha, you seems to have done a good job in helping Mike to contain his anger. We think you should continue to do so until Jane leaves. Or, it may be too hard on Mike if his anger blows.
>
> MCBRIDE: Maybe you could rehearse or practice. You know how to deal with Jane's difficulties. Before "the right time" comes, use her next crisis to rehearse expressing your feelings and anticipating her reactions.

On the way out of the room, Mr. Jay again remarked that Martha may fall apart if Jane moves out. As they were heading down the front steps, they were given another tag:

> MCBRIDE: Steve says that thinking about the worst may be too anxiety provoking for both of you.

Study Efforts

The team had observed Mike and Martha nodding several times during the message, in particular at the mention of "rehearsing." The team predicted that Mike and Martha would give Jane the message, including the deadline. They also predicted that Jane would "raise hell," which might be described as continuing to sacrifice herself, particularly if she perceives that her parents need her help to stay together. The team also predicted that Martha and Mike would continue to enjoy each other more as they continued to perceive their situation differently and thus behave differently.

Session 4

As the session begins, Mike asks Derks and McBride how *they* have been getting along since the last session:

> DERKS: Oh, just fine. We're getting along much better.
> *(The phone rings.)*
> DERKS: Steve disagrees!

All four of them laughed, and the session continued to be rather light and humorous. Martha had a new hairdo and appeared more relaxed than during any previous session.

Mr. and Mrs. Jay reported giving the message to Jane and that they had found her an apartment several blocks away. Jane surprised them by agreeing to move, and so they saw no need for a deadline. They were prepared for any reaction except the one they received. However, the next day Jane got fired from her job. When mother heard this, she clapped. At this point, Mr. and Mrs. Jay considered extending their original deadline, although they had not as yet given Jane *any* deadline:

> *(The phone rings.)*
> DERKS: Steve wonders: Now that Jane undermined the deadline, now what? She could be without a job until she's twenty-seven.
> MR. JAY: If she gets unemployment, she still has to move.
> DERKS: What if no job, no unemployment?
> MRS. JAY: She'll get it.
> DERKS: Then the deadline still holds.
> MRS. JAY: If we don't, we're failing her, keeping her still a child.

They agreed to inform Jane that she has a deadline, one that is two weeks after the original one they had planned.

Jane's getting fired is in line with the predictions: She is continuing to behave as though to sacrifice herself until her parents prove to her that they no longer need her to help them stay together. However, Martha and Mike did give the message together, and they did not back down when Jane got fired. This is a good sign that Martha and Mike are perceiving things differently. Martha did not develop any symptoms, and she did not behave as though to protect Jane from the dangers of moving out, and neither did Mike. Including the deadline with the original message would have been preferable since it would have given Jane a stronger message about parental unity.

Junior was now getting ready to come out of the hospital and had requested permission for he and his wife to come and live with the senior Jays until they got back on their feet. Mike and Martha rejected this request.

It is almost predictable that one of the children will react to Martha's and Mike's changes by attempting to act as if keeping mother and father together. Junior may even perceive things in such a way that he may need to "act crazy" again if he thinks his parents need that kind of sacrifice.

The remainder of the session was spent comparing how Mr. and Mrs. Jay had adjusted to things their children did and how they were able to accept these "new things," whereas the children did not accept new things the parents did.

The Jays went on to describe how their elderly parents were able to accept change better than their children.

Consulting Break

The primary concern was that Martha might again get depressed or have some somatic symptoms, or that Jane might get around the deadline, or that Junior might return to the nest, or Joan might return, or Junior might act crazy. The team decided to build the compliment around the changes made and build the clue around the concerns.

Message Giving

> DERKS: We're all struck by your ability to make changes, which causes us to doubt the old cliche about "you can't teach old dogs new tricks." It looks like it's the young dogs who can't change. Our concern is that Jane and Junior have already learned to fly.
>
> McBRIDE: It does seem to us that the kids have already learned to fly, but they just don't know it yet. You've seen it, but they don't realize they've done it.

On the way down the stairs, McBride finished the intervention as a tag.

> McBRIDE: Steve reminded me of an old saying: "If you let the camel get his nose in the tent, pretty soon you'll have the whole camel in the tent." *(The Jays laughed.)*

Study Efforts

The team predicted that Martha and Mike would deliver and enforce the deadline and that they would stick to their decision not to allow Mike Jr. to return to the nest. Furthermore, the team predicted that Martha would be even less depressed and that Mike's "lip would be less stiff."

Session 5

Two weeks later the fifth session again opened with humor, as Martha and Mike played around with deciding who was going to start:

> MRS. JAY: Things are coming along quite well, as far as the kids go. I'm doing very well!

DERKS: Did the camel get the nose in the tent?
MRS. JAY: No. The camel is home, living with his wife.

The extended deadline for Jane's move was still in the future. Jane did not yet have a job nor did she get unemployment. However, she was drinking less, and her boyfriend had a job for the first time in months, which stabilized their situation.

Early in the interval between sessions, Mike started to feel depressed. At first he was not sure why since he saw three possible reasons. When he discussed it with Martha, they narrowed it down to his work situation. During their talk it became clear to him that he still had the option of changing jobs and he would then feel less trapped. One of the main difficulties on the job was with a coworker, a recovering alcoholic who was much younger than Mike. Mike was very supportive of his attempt to stop drinking and was conscientious in helping to build up his coworker.

The team was well aware that, for the third session in a row, Martha was not showing depressed feelings and she was not complaining about somatic symptoms. The goals named in the first session were essentially achieved.

The Jays were now dealing with each other directly, and together they were dealing with some of those "damn things" that constitute life. They were not allowing the children's problems to interfere.

Consulting Break

The team decided that Mike's difficulty at work was a worthwhile issue for the Jays to be dealing with at this point. Since it was an issue they could do something about and they were dealing with it appropriately, this concern needed to be built into the intervention. A further emphasis needed was for Mr. and Mrs. Jay to address their teamwork to solving their problems rather than the kids' problems.

Message Giving

DERKS: We were really impressed with how methodically you two have gone about solving this problem. Both of you know, the battle's half-won once you've identified what the problem is and prioritized it as you've done.

McBRIDE: I guess I was thinking too, that the kids' not causing you a problem left you free to deal with your own problems.

MR. JAY: And Jane has not been any problem.

DERKS: You've got some good plans for continuing to get out of the depression.

MR. JAY: Yeah.

DERKS: Steve had another point thought, too. He wasn't sure he agreed with your idea that your partner is helping you out and was thinking you may be helping him out, especially around this recovering alcoholic business. He needs to build himself up.

MR. JAY: I go along with that.

DERKS: And, you're not denying him that. You're almost sacrificing yourself so that he can build himself up at times.

MR. JAY: That might be on my mind. I'm sixty. I see this guy's really got a battle, and I figure: If I can help him win this battle, I'm all for it.

McBRIDE: So, actually you've got two counselors in the family now.

Study Effort

Throughout the message, Martha and Mike smiled and nodded. The team's job was to keep the Jays outside of their original frame and to help them to continue to work as a unit: a behavioral change that indicates a perceptual change on both parts. It is noteworthy that Martha did not get depressed or develop somatic symptoms when Mike started to feel depressed: She did not take over and carry the burden for him since he had "loosened up his lips" enough to talk to her about this situation.

The team predicted Martha would not experience either depression or somatic symptoms. The team predicted that Mike's depression would disappear. Further, the team predicted more joint activities, even if the children experienced new difficulties. Jane's moving would be the signal to the team to terminate therapy.

Session 6

The sixth session centered around a "little tiff" Martha and Mike had several days before. During the argument, Martha expressed her anger, punched a kitchen cabinet, and went for a fast walk about the block. Both of them were glad this had happened because the new elements served to convince them "things were really different." After she returned from the walk, they discussed the incident. Mike had been afraid throughout that Martha would hyperventilate; but she did not. Mike had also been worried about her blood pressure getting higher, which did not happen. Both considered these good signs.

Furthermore, neither of them got depressed. Finally, since they had not had many arguments that did not revolve around the kids, they were pleased that they were able to talk things out and discover that "making up" after the fight was the best part.

Jane had found a job, and her moving deadline was less than a week away. She seemed to like the job and was drinking even less. They had told Jane that once she moved, she would not be moving back.

The rest of the session was devoted to their plans for adjusting to being a "young married couple" again. They could now fix up their house to suit them, and they could travel more freely.

Consulting Break

The argument was further confirmation that the Jays had broken out of the original frame and thus were perceiving things differently and were behaving differently: no symptoms, no depression, no stiff upper lip, no children involved. They were standing on their own feet.

All of these changes were apparent; the team decided to address these changes in the message and to stop therapy at this point except for a follow-up session in one month.

Message Giving

DERKS: We were impressed with the way you, Martha, handled the anger. It sounds like a real healthy way. Obviously, letting it out is a much better way than holding it in and ending up hyperventilating.

MRS. JAY: Yeah, for sure.

DERKS: Or, other psychosomatic stuff.

MRS. JAY: That psychosomatic stuff is really scary.

DERKS: We are also impressed with the way you, Mike, handled it, too. We were surprised that you didn't hold some sort of grudge, but you got right back in there and settled it with her.

MR. JAY: I was really worried about the hyperventilating, so even expressing the anger didn't upset me.

DERKS: It seems, too, that you're both on the right track with Jane and the other "camel." Perhaps it's time to call off the "therapy dogs." Things are going well with you two. I want to warn you that, over the next couple of weeks, with Jane gone, it might be a bit of a crisis time. And there might be some kind of a relapse.

Study Effort

In the team's opinion, the Jays were working well enough as a unit and the perceptual-behavioral changes were "stable enough" that therapy could stop. The team predicted that either Jane's acting up or Junior's acting crazy would not cause Martha and Mike to go back to the old frame. Although the team might have preferred to have Jane's move completed before stopping therapy, the move was not part of the original goals-signs.

Follow-Up

Jane had moved out and was successful in holding her job. Junior had taken on a larger apartment house to manage so he and his wife had moved a couple of miles away. Neither Martha nor Mike had any complaints. Both were dieting, and she had applied for a new full-time job.

Contact with the Jays six months later indicated that the frame was firmly in place. None of the old complaints had recurred.

CHAPTER 8

The Jones Family

The therapy of the Jones family presented in this chapter differs from the Jay family's therapy of previous chapter in several ways. Unlike the Jay family, the Jones family was never able to define a specific goal for the therapy, which makes it difficult for the family and the team to know success or failure when the therapy stops. The Jones family's type of vagueness was a significant part of its pattern and the way it showed its manner of cooperating, and, therefore, vagueness was a significant part of the way the team was able to cooperate.

Twice during the therapy the team gave the family copies of the intervention the conductor (de Shazer) read to the family. These typed interventions were given to the family to help it focus on the tasks of therapy and to help it change through the use of an "interspersal technique" of imbedding suggestions for change within a larger context. Erickson constructed the prototype, which involves some peculiar sentence construction, such as, "I wonder if the tomato plant can, Joe, feel really feel a kind of comfort" (35, p. 517). In a conversation that appears to be about a tomato plant, Erickson interspersed the real message (underscored), which he indicated with a change of voice and pauses. The use of this technique with a "vague" family allows the conductor to "appear" to be as vague and as confused as the family, while it also allows him to focus on the change the family desires. The real message (which is underscored) is embedded among other, insignificant words. For instance: "If you were to (pause) Mrs. Jones, stop being bitchy, that might upset your family." The therapeutic suggestion ("Mrs. Jones stop being bitchy"), set off by pauses, is interspersed within a context of telling her not to stop. The conductor changes his tone of voice while giving the suggestion. Frequently enough, the party follows through on the suggestions. Giving the same messages in note form seemed to be effective with this family.

A CASE STUDY

During the initial phone call Mrs. Jones informed us that the school psychologist had suggested therapy for the family. Her son, Robert (aged 15), was

130

uncooperative both at home and at school, where he was not doing well. The family had been in therapy before, but after one joint session, the previous therapist saw them individually or in pairs. Mrs. Jones did not like this because it allowed for secrets. Her idea was that therapy meant "letting it all hang out." Things had been no better after this attempt.

Presession Planning

Prior to the first session the team* met to develop a temporary map to guide the conductor's explorations. The team suspected that Sarah Jones was "overinvolved" with her son, Robert, and that Robert's uncooperativeness was as attempt to become less involved with mother. She, therefore, became more intrusive, which was followed by more uncooperativeness. Father's part was unknown, and the team suspected there might be some distance between father and mother. It should be noted that this wording of the map is not very *useful* since it is not positive. It might, however, be accurate and truthful.

Another map was developed that was more useful. The team suspected that Robert's uncooperativeness might be seen as protective of his parents, aimed at keeping them together. Certainly Robert's behavior at home and at school gave the parents something in common, something to talk to each other about. The team (aware that when asked for a two sentence description of the problem, Mrs. Jones had talked for 25 minutes) suspected that Mrs. Jones' "overwhelming number of words" might protect Mr. Jones from having to deal with the boy's problems. Furthermore, her words might protect father from the boy in some ways. The team preferred the second map because it was more positive and more useful.

The team also wondered what "secrets" Mrs. Jones might fear and if these same problems had been evident before Robert entered high school, where he was in a "learning-impaired" class.

Prelude to Session 1

When the Jones family arrived, the conductor explained about the mirror and the videotaping and that the team would be behind the mirror. He also explained that after 40 minutes, he would consult with the team and would share with the family what the team said.

Sam Jones (aged 52) had been employed for many years at the same job, which he enjoyed. Sarah Jones (aged 54) was employed part-time with the

---

*In addition to de Shazer, the team included Alex Molnar and Jo Ellyn Schultz (both were then graduate students). In subsequent sessions, Insoo Berg and Jim Derks joined the team.

school system. Robert was in the ninth grade at a four-year high school, which he did not enjoy. They described the neighborhood as deteriorating over the 20 years during which they had lived in the same house. They did not practice any religion and did not seem to be involved in the neighborhood. Robert was the only child.

Data Collecting

DE SHAZER: Well, what problem can we help you with?

MRS. JONES: I went to a school conference and I had an appointment with the psychologist. Bobby had seen her, the way I understood it when he left [his previous school], she'd see him more frequently. I thought I'd stop in, she didn't have much time, but she talked to me when he went to [elementary school] she was at that school at that time.

I said, "The problem's the same, you know." She said, "Well, I won't be seeing Bobby so often, because"—can I say this? She said, "If Bobby ever feels like," when he went to [his previous school], he saw Mr. ah . . .

ROBERT: Thorton.

MRS. JONES: Mr. Thorton twice a week and she said she wouldn't be seeing Bobby that often. Bobby has a tendency—which is true—to create, ah, well, more problems than he really has. But he should feel that if he ever really has a problem, she's there. We were going to Dr. Zarkov for a while, and I went to school—maybe things at home were a little better, not terrific—but Dr. Zarkov said we were improving. She said we were improving, but I couldn't see it. Could you?

MR. JONES: Ah . . . no.

MRS. JONES: *(Overlapping the "no.")* Then I went to school—I could have rented a room at that school—his one teacher had him for two semesters. I can't remember. Name his name.

ROBERT: Mrs. Bello?

MRS. JONES: No, the one with the glasses. English teacher. Name her.

ROBERT: Mrs. White.

MRS. JONES: That's the one. I went to see her and I said, "How's Bobby doing?" "Errr." *(Mrs. Jones demonstrated pulling her hair.)* I said, "Oh, you poor thing."

Mother's monologue continued in a similar fashion for 15 more minutes. The conductor tried to interrupt on several occasions without success. Words alone were not sufficient. Finally, the conductor was able to stem the tide by holding up his hand in the "stop-sign" fashion which arrested the flow. The conductor attempted to help the family focus on current complaints, but his efforts were rewarded with more details about the history of the problem and the efforts Mrs. Jones had made to get school psychologists, social workers, and therapists to really help. At several points Mrs. Jones was stuck for a word or a detail, and either Sam or Robert would fill it in with little or no problem. Mrs. Jones would immediately resume her story.

Once the conductor was able to get the family to focus on the current complaints, a wealth of issues appeared. Both Mr. and Mrs. Jones complained that Bobby mumbled and swore a lot under his breath. They further complained that Bobby was not doing well in school, getting a lot of "D" grades and failures. Mr. Jones did recount one major exception in shop class two years earlier when Bobby had received an "A." Neither the parents nor the school thought Bobby was working up to his potential. Mrs. Jones further complained that Bobby did not hang up his clothes, make his bed, or keep his room sufficiently clean. And, Bobby did not know the value of money, and, therefore, he always wanted more expensive things than they could afford. They also complained that once he got these things, he would only use them for a short while.

Goals. The Jones family wanted to see Bobby's attitude change because neither parent thought Bobby respected them as parents. Mrs. Jones then continued onto school improvements, less swearing, better control of his temper, less mumbling under his breath, hanging up his clothes, and so on. Bobby wanted his mother to holler at him less. The conductor made efforts to help them focus on one significant change, but they were unable to decide which was most important. Each thing mentioned led to further things and more details.

The team observed that Mrs. Jones was very concerned and was really working hard at getting professional help. It seemed certain that Bobby saw mother's involvement as a "positive." It seemed that Mr. Jones worked hard and that he was patient, accepting, and quiet. He did not seem "withdrawn"; rather he seemed involved in a quiet way since he did know what was going on in the family and was able to help out his wife with details. When directly asked a question, he responded with more clarity than did Mrs. Jones.

Consulting Break

The team speculated that Bobby's "uncooperativeness" allowed, or made it possible for, his parents to be involved with him. His behavior certainly seemed to bring them together on his issues. His behavior also taught the parents how to be patient in dealing with various professionals. It also seemed that Bobby was behaving as though he was protecting his parents from some problem(s) between them.

Mrs. Jones showed that giving details and reporting on incidents was her way of cooperating with the therapy. Mr. Jones and Robert showed their way of cooperating with her in this was by not interrupting. Furthermore, unlike the tendency among the team members, Sam and Robert did not tune out her monologue.

The family's approach to its problems seemed to focus on mother's efforts, and the reports of these efforts were rather perplexing since she interspersed "data" among other details and comments. The goals were not clearly established, and no signs were developed.

The team decided to compliment the family on the way it behaved during the first part of the session. That is, the team attempted to reframe the family's way of cooperating as shown so far. Since the family was at least unfocused and it had broadly painted its picture of the situation, the team decided to give it a message that was as vague and general. The team wanted the family to have a success with the task and hoped that it would be more focused in the next session.

Since Mrs. Jones could be described as using an "interspersal technique," the team used the same technique in the message to Mr. Jones.

Message Giving

DE SHAZER: We are impressed, really impressed (*facing Robert*) with how open and clear you all are about these complex issues. We were particularly struck with the way you, Robert, are so open, which (*facing Mrs. Jones*) we find to be unusual with adolescents. We are very impressed, Mr. Jones, with your patience in these matters. We know how hard it is for a person of your type, the strong silent type not to blow up, even when they think it might be necessary.

MRS. JONES: He doesn't like to fight.

DE SHAZER: We are also impressed with your ability to give detailed and full descriptions, Mrs. Jones.

Between now and next time we meet, we would like all three of you to think about what you do *not* want to see change about how you each get along with the others.

All three agreed to do the task, and Mrs. Jones continued to mutter the instructions under her breath while they were leaving the room.

Study Effort

The team predicted that the Jones family would keep the next scheduled appointment. As is frequently the case with first-session interventions, the clue was just aimed at "seeing what they will do with it." Since the family's goals were so broad and so wide in scope that they became vague, the team's clue was appropriately vague and broad. Although the team hoped this clue would help the Jones family focus more either by developing a list of things not to change or by concentrating on one particular thing to change, neither of these was the main purpose of the clue. The main purpose of the clue, particularly in first sessions, is just to discover how the family will show its unique way of cooperating.

The compliment set of the intervention was broadly isomorphic with the patterns the family showed the team during the main part of the session. Mrs. Jones gave the team full and detailed descriptions, Robert was quite open and clear, and Mr. Jones was quiet. The imbedded suggestion (that Mr. Jones' silence was an attempt to not blow up, even though he might think it necessary) was also an experiment to test that style of communication with the family. Since the team described Mr. Jones as a careful listener and Mrs. Jones as using an interspersal technique, it designed this message in an attempt to be isomorphic with that part of the family pattern. The team also predicted that Mr. Jones *might* do something more active about his complaints.

Session 2

DE SHAZER: Well, how has the week been?

MRS. JONES: Don't ask.

MR. JONES: Rough.

MRS. JONES: Same thing.

(Pause.)

DE SHAZER: We asked you to think about what you do not want to see change.

MRS. JONES: Does that mean the things we want to stay the same?

DE SHAZER: OK.

MR. JONES: I mulled that over in my mind a million times.

ROBERT: *(Interrupting.)* Me, too.

MR. JONES: I can't think of a thing, really.

ROBERT: That's how I got this headache.

MRS. JONES: I don't want anything to stay the way it is.

MR. JONES: There isn't a thing I can think of I want to stay the same.

MRS. JONES: I'm saying the same thing you are.

(Pause.)

MR. JONES: At the supper table last night, and it's not only last night, it's every night: He's up and down, up and down. And you gotta tell him, "Bob, sit down. Eat your supper."

DE SHAZER: When he gets up, what does he do when he's up?

MR. JONES: Goes to his room; goes to the bathroom; goes to the living room.

DE SHAZER: Doing what?

MR. JONES: He goes to his bedroom to play with his kittens. Of course, if he goes to the bathroom, I can see that.

The team was greatly surprised when Mr. Jones initiated the complaints and when he continued to talk without interruption or assistance from either Mrs. Jones or Robert. During this speech the team observed Mrs. Jones to be carefully watching and listening to Mr. Jones, often nodding when he made a point.

Mr. Jones went on to describe an incident the previous evening. He had given Robert a job to perform, but Robert did not do it. Mr. Jones asked "Why not?" He never got a satisfactory response. Mr. Jones complained about this behavior but did nothing further. He and Mrs. Jones went onto complain about how frequently they had to holler at Robert. Mrs. Jones thought that if she could holler less, then there would be more harmony around the house.

Mrs. Jones complained that all the hollering left her feeling bitchy and that bitchiness was effecting her work performance. Mr. Jones then complained about how often they both had to call Robert when supper was ready.

Robert's main complaint was that his mother called him repeatedly to get him up in the morning. He claimed that he was awake and her calling "bugged" him. Bob also complained that his father has "come off like Al Capone" during the week, which meant that he gave Bob orders rather than requests.

When the conductor attempted to narrow down any of these complaints in order to develop a goal or a sign of progress, Mr. and/or Mrs. Jones would quickly deny the significance of that particular "sign" and then explore some other aspect of Robert's behavior.

Consulting Break

The team was pleased to see the relatively more focused session and the switch in word distribution between Mr. and Mrs. Jones. It wondered if there were an interconnection between the message in the first session and Mr. Jones "coming off like Al Capone" and talking more in the second session.

All three had performed the task: thinking about what *not* to change. However, their thoughts seemed to go in the opposite direction: thinking about what *to* change. The second session produced little or no improvement in the focus or goal directedness, except that the complaints in the session centered around the supper hour. It seemed clear that the family responded to the vague first session clue and the interspersed suggestion. The team decided that a task that calls for a behavior change around the supper hour might give more information about the Jones family's manner of cooperating.

Message Giving

> DE SHAZER: We've all been impressed with the ability all of you have to think clearly, and not only to think clearly, but to put those thoughts into words. A lot of people we work with cannot quite do that anywhere near as well as you three seem to be able to do. So, our picture of what's going on is getting clearer.
>
> Now, what we'd like you to do between now and next time we meet is, we's like each of you—all three of you—to do *something different*, once during the week, either before or during the supper hour. Just as an experiment to see what happens.

All three agreed after Mr. Jones repeated the task.

Study Effort

The team predicted that the Jones family would return and would have found some way to react to the experiment other than ignore it. The team predicted that the response report would be vague and the data interspersed within other contexts. The team did not expect the shift in word distribution to continue into the next session.

Session 3

Mr. Jones and Robert both stated that they were unable to think of anything different to do before or during the supper hour. Mrs. Jones decided immediately after the previous session to call Robert only one time each day for supper, and she stuck to that throughout the week. Despite Mr. Jones' saying he could not think of anything to do, he did not call Robert for supper throughout the week. Robert, despite his disclaimer, came to supper after having been called only once each day, and he was not late for any suppers.

During the session Mr. Jones complained about coming home to the "same old thing day after day." Everyday he came home to hear complaints about Robert and to find more things about which to complain.

Robert had a run-in with the police when he arrived late for school. He was able to control his temper and, with the assistance of school personnel, he was able to work out this situation without the involvement of his mother.

As usual, the specific information was buried in a wealth of other information, and the conductor had to use careful questioning to elicit the responses to the task.

Consulting Break

The task response report conformed to the idea the team had about the family's manner of cooperating. This method of reporting by interspersing the data among other information and the denials can be seen as reasonable for a family that wants to change everything. Anything less than everything is seen as insignificant. Another point seemed significant to the team: The task called for doing something different *once,* and all three members of the family had carried that to an extreme by doing the same "different" thing everyday. The team wondered if this exaggeration was also another part of the family pattern that went along with the idea of "changing everything."

During the session the team developed a written intervention or message. The team thought that the Jones family would respond to vague messages that followed this pattern: They could change while continuing to deny the change. By using the interspersal technique, the team could continue to cooperate with the Jones family's manner of cooperating, and the team could be isomorphic by telling it to change within a larger context of telling them not to change. In this way the team's message would fit the family patterns and its way of cooperating because the total message would be vague but it would include the significant information buried among other words. The suggestions interspersed in the context will be <u>underscored</u>, and the *pauses* will be indicated. The copies given to the Jones family did not include these "stage directions."

The team also decided to build a compliment around the parents' difficulty in coming home and the boy's manner of handling the incident with the police. Each of these, of course, were described from a different angle.

Message Giving

> DE SHAZER: We are surprised that—since you know what you're going home to—that you're willing to go right home. Most guys would probably make a long stop at a bar.
>
> MRS. JONES: We don't drink, but I've also thought about running away.
>
> DE SHAZER: And, we're surprised, Mrs. Jones, that you don't meet him in the bar. Also, we are surprised that you [Robert] handled the episode with the cops so well. I remember being your age and feeling hassled by the cops, and I think I would have lost control of my temper.

We've thought a lot about your situation, and I'm going to read you our ideas.

We know that you'd like to (*pause*) Mrs. Jones stop being bitchy and (*pause*) stop hollering at Bob (*pause*) but we don't think that would be a wise idea right now because you need to continue trying to teach Bob to be responsible for himself (*pause*) and that's the best way you've found. If you were to (*pause*) Mrs. Jones stop hollering right now, that might upset the balance of your family in some way.

And, we know that there are times when you'd like to (*pause*) Mr. Jones come off like Al Capone (*pause*) but we are afraid that if you were to do that, then it might upset the balance of your family: Neither your wife nor your son would like it. We think that you need to continue to *act* like the "strong silent type" because neither Bob nor your wife would like it if you did most of the hollering or if you were to (*pause*) Mr. Jones often come off like Al Capone.

We realize that you'd be better off if you were to (*pause*) Bob have a better attitude (*pause*) stop calling people names and (*pause*) Bob stop mumbling to yourself under your breath. But, adolescents —like you—need to rebel in some way, like being difficult to get up in the morning. It might make life easier for you to (*pause*) Bob get up when called (*pause*) and continue (*pause*) to come to supper when when called, but then your mother and father would be likely to wonder what you're up to next. We think you cause them more than enough worry right now without adding to it by (*puase*) getting up quickly in the morning and (*pause*) coming to the table quickly.

So, at this point, I think we should be very, very cautious about changing things; moving very, very slowly. We'd like you to take along copies and think about it and read it once or twice between now and next session.

Study Effort

Mrs. Jones was observed to nod several times during her section of the message, particularly at the very end when the team used her phrase "upset the balance of your family." Both Mr. and Mrs. Jones nodded and smiled at the suggestion that Mr. Jones might do most of the hollering. Throughout father's section, Bob was seen to squirm, particularly during the two references to "Al Capone." Bob nodded when all three suggestions were given in the first sentence of his section and again during the repeats. Mother and father also nodded during Robert's section.

The team thought that the interspersed suggestions would be effective because of the isomorphism between the message and the family's patterns, as the team had described these patterns. The message built on the interspersal technique should be familiar to the family, and, therefore, this message shows that the team is cooperating with the family's demonstrated manner of cooperating.

Each of the suggestions was aimed at complaints the family had mentioned in the three sessions. The team predicted that the Jones family would report some changes in the morning complaint, the supper complaint, and the hollering complaint. The team also predicted that Mr. Jones would act more forcefully about something during the interval.

Since the family goal was to "change everything," the team would ultimately have to decide when to stop therapy. If this intervention were successful in changing the complaint areas, then these changes might be sufficient signs of progress.

Session 4

During the two weeks Robert only had to be called once in the morning, and on three days he was up before being called. Each day he made his bed. Except for one day of the period, Robert continued to need to be called only once for supper. Mother found herself feeling less bitchy.

One school night Bob wanted special permission to go out with his friends and to stay out much later than his parents would usually allow. Frequently in the past either Robert would have been able to talk them into this permission or he would have been able to divide the parents and would go without permission. This time his parents "put their heads together" and did not allow themselves to be talked into it or to be divided. Robert stayed home even though he mumbled and swore about it.

One day father complained about Bob's playing his music too loudly after he had tolerated it for two hours. Bob refused to either turn it down or off. Sam hit Bob for the first time in years, and shortly after the music was off. The parents saw this as a failure since Bob had not complied with the request immediately, and father did not connect his hitting Bob with the result. However, this was not what concerned Mr. and Mrs. Jones most at this time.

Most of the fourth session was devoted to Bob's desire to have a pellet gun. Father was determined to stand firmly against it because he and Mrs. Jones worried about how Robert might misuse the gun. Robert was sure that he could talk his father into it within an hour and a half. Mrs. Jones reported that this was the usual way things went: Eventually, Bob would talk his father into it, or he would talk his mother into it, and they would join forces to talk Mr. Jones into it.

Consulting Break

The pellet gun discussion was the first clear report of a specific pattern involving all three members of the family. All of them agreed that history was likely to repeat, and the team saw this as a key pattern to the situation. Therefore, the team decided to attempt to modify the outcome of this pattern. In keeping with the family's style, the third alternative would be suggested in the middle of the two that the family predicted.

Message Giving

DE SHAZER: Well, we were all really surprised and pleased at your determination to protect Bob on Sunday [the music incident] and not really come off like Al Capone—even though part of you felt like it.

And, we were surprised that you, Mrs. Jones, were able to stay out of it as well as you did. That's really good.

We were pleased to hear that you [Robert] cleaned up your bike and your Dad's bike without ever being asked.

Now, we have some homework for you: Sometime between now and next time we meet, Bob and Dad, I want you Bob to spend one and a half hours trying to talk your Dad into this gun thing. During that time, while they are doing this, we suggest you [Mrs. Jones] go out for a walk or something: Let them handle this.

Now, we have some bets. We were split even on this, so I don't know. (Pause.) Some of us are betting that you're [Mr. Jones] going to give in. And some of us are betting that you won't give in. The third bet is that you're [Mrs. Jones] going to help Bob talk Dad into it. So, we'll find out next time who wins.

Study Effort

At this point, the team predicted that father's Al Capone part was strong enough to pick the new alternative—not giving in. The other two choices were the family's predicted outcomes. By naming all three options, the team would be cooperating with whatever response the family might report.

Comment. It is interesting to note that the family seemed to become more specific in this session. The team has to assume that the intervention in the previous session interconnects with this change as well as with the changes in the morning complaint, the supper complaint, and the hollering complaint. In reaction to this shift by the family, the team follows along and gives the family a concrete task. That is, when the family's response report indicates a concrete response to a vague task, then the team switches to a more concrete type of clue. The circularity of the decision tree (Chapter 4) is meant to guide the team in this switch.

Since the design of interventions is guided by the concurrent concepts of cooperating and isomorphism, this switch can also be described as a method of making sure the intervention design is isomorphic. By telling the family to go ahead with its usual pattern and suggesting a new outcome, the team is using the suggested new outcome to create the different angle. Thus, Bob may get the idea that Dad will not be talked into the gun; and Dad will get the idea that he does not have to allow himself to be talked into the gun; and Mother may get the idea that Dad will not be talked into the gun. A new pattern may emerge.

Session 5

(Mrs. Jones called before the session to report she was ill and she wondered if it would be OK if just Bob and his father came.)

Mr. Jones had not given in about the gun, and now Robert was not sure that he even wanted one. Therefore, he had not spent any time trying to talk his father into it. Mr. Jones was convinced that he would not allow himself to be talked into it.

The changes already made in the morning complaint, the supper complaint, and the hollering complaint had continued, and this was for a three-week interval since session 4.

The conductor worried about what the parents would find to worry about next. Mr. Jones provided the answer—school. Mr. Jones and Robert spent most of the session talking about what was going on at school. Mr. Jones stated his opinions in a very firm manner.

Consulting Break

Given Mrs. Jones' worries about secrets, the team took the change of her sending Mr. Jones and Robert as a sign of progress and as confirmation that her perceptions were changing and, therefore, that she could behave differently.

Because the previous written message seemed so effective and because of Mrs. Jones' concerns for secrets, the team prepared another message.

Message Giving

DE SHAZER: We've done it again. We've thought about things and have another message for you.

When thinking about and reviewing our last meeting, we became concerned about several things: (*1*) Bob, we worried about your getting up after being called only once during a whole two weeks, and now it's five weeks, because we don't think you—his parents—need the extra worry about what Bob might be up to next. For the same reason, we worried about you—his parents—having to call Bob only once for supper each day. (*2*) We were puzzled about your teamwork when you put your heads together about not giving Bob that special permission that one evening. Like Bob, we are worried about you two coming off like Bonnie and Clyde—who were famous for working well together as a team. We don't think you two—Mom and Dad—should (*pause*) come off like Bonnie and Clyde—because it would change things too quickly, and it might really upset the balance of your family. (*3*) We think your swearing and mumbling under your breath is probably a good idea for right now because it helps you to—Bobby control your temper. If you—Bobby stop swearing and mumbling under your breath, you'll probably lose your temper more often.

We have copies of that for you.

Study Effort

The team predicted more team work and less swearing and mumbling as well as the continuation of the previous changes.

The team decided to return to the vague, interspersal technique because the report on the previous task was unclear. Although Mr. Jones had not yet been talked into the gun, Bobby had not yet given it a real try. Now, the team could have described this as a successful intervention since Bob's behavior could be an indication that he had the idea that Dad was not going to be talked into the pellet gun. The team predicted Bob would renew his efforts to talk Dad into the gun. The previous intervention had been successful in terms of the scope of any intervention holding for only the interval between sessions: Dad indeed did not allow himself to be talked into the gun.

Session 6

Bob had received a "B" in each of four subjects; he had received a "B" for conduct in all of his classes except one in which he received an "A."

DE SHAZER: I believe it, but I don't understand it. This could be a real problem. Now they'll expect you to get "A"s and "B"s all the time. This could really upset the balance.

The conductor suggested that the report card might be "the thing" that really upset the balance. Father agreed that the shock of Bob's report card might upset the balance in an unfavorable way, though he also agreed with Mrs. Jones that a favorable change was possible. The family reported continued changes, including less swearing and mumbling.

Mr. Jones wondered how we were going to settle our bet because the outcome was not any of those choices bet upon. Bob had found a way to get the pellet gun from one of his uncles. Mr. and Mrs. Jones were upset, but they put their heads together and came up with specific rules. If Bob violated any of those rules, even once, then he would lose the gun.

Consulting Break

The team saw this outcome as yet another vague response. Bobby seemed convinced he could not talk Dad into the gun, and so he went around the block. On the other hand, Mother and Dad were pulling together and had set firm, concrete rules for the use of the gun.

The report card seemed a significant indication that there was a major change in the family system. Bob's school behavior seemed to indictate a change in his perceptions, and the parents (and the school) needed to respond to that change.

Message Giving

DE SHAZER: We think you were wise in deciding to go slow about the gun thing, and not making a big issue of it because if you had dropped it in the river, that would have upset the balance in the wrong direction.

One thing that struck us was your [Mr. and Mrs. Jones] continuing to want to take on this big project of changing the balance of your family. And, you have been thinking a lot about that, I gather. Again, we continue to caution you about moving too fast.

We are certainly impressed that you [Robert] were smart enough to have hidden your intelligence up to now, and we are further struck by the fact you didn't get too high conduct grades, because that would have really been too hard to live up to.

Now, we know that you two [Mr. and Mrs. Jones] are interested in changing this balance in a favorable direction. We think you two should talk to each other about this and decide when it is the right time to do this so you don't upset the balance in an unfavorable direction. For instance, we think you're going to run into misuse of the gun, and we think you should plan your approach to this. We suggest that you go for a walk, or at least make sure that these talks are not heard by Bob.

Study Effort

The team predicted more teamwork and that Bob would misuse the gun sometime in the month-long interval. The team also predicted that Mr. and Mrs. Jones would stand firm about the gun issue once Bob misused it and that the changes already made would stick.

Session 7

DE SHAZER: You've had several weeks now since Bob got those "B"s and "A"s in conduct. How has that upset things? We've worried a lot about that.

MRS. JONES: They may put him into a higher track of classes.

DE SHAZER: So, it may upset the balance over there, in school instead of at home?

MR. JONES: I never thought about that, but that's a real possibility.

Mrs. Jones went on to describe the teamwork and that Bob had not misused the pellet gun at all during the month. She had had to holler less, and she thought Bob was swearing less. The previous reported changes were sticking.

Consulting Break

The team's hunch that this would be the last session was confirmed. The family seemed to be behaving differently, and it seemed to be handling those differences.

The team decided to terminate with some more clues. It was necessary to remember that the Jones family wanted "nothing to stay the same." Therefore, it might perceive the changes it described as not truly significant. Yet, from the team's perspective, the changes were significant. More time was needed to see if the changes were eventually perceived as significant by Mr. and Mrs. Jones.

Message Giving

DE SHAZER: Well, we were all thinking about this and remembering when you first came in that you all three wanted nothing to remain the same. Which is sort of a "mission impossible task." And, of course,

Bob's going to swear and mumble—most boys his age do—and we think it prevents him from losing his temper more often than he does. And, as long as he swears and mumbles, you two are in no danger of having to learn how to live with a saint.

And, you're right in thinking that I was really shocked about the grades. We all were. And, we were afraid it was going to upset things at home. And it might not. What it might do is upset things at school. But, we don't know yet. So, we'd like to suggest at this point that we stop today, see how things go. Let me know if the balance gets unfavorably upset at home. We may have helped you change too many things: We just have to wait and see. Maybe see what the grades are like next time.

Follow-Up

At the end of six months, the family had not yet called. When the family was contacted, it was discovered that Robert's grades had held up through two more marking periods and that Robert still had not misused the pellet gun. The changes made during therapy had held up.

When the new school year started, Robert was placed in a higher track, and, according to the school psychologist, he continued to perform well. He had received "A"s and "B"s in both course work and conduct.

CHAPTER 9

Complexity

In the preceding chapters, various descriptive tools have been used to explicate the binocular theory of change and the methods used to implement the theory. The multiple explanations and descriptions of the same processes follow Bateson's notion that two (or more) descriptions of the same processes provide more depth—some sort of "bonus." We hope that this bonus will be some useful ideas about family therapy and the processes of change.

As the therapy with each family, couple, or individual, develops, any, or better all, of the maps are useful. The balance theoretical maps (Chapter 6) help the therapist focus on the goal directedness of therapy. It is only with goals in mind that the therapist and the family can *know* that therapy is successful. Even when the family has been unable to focus or articulate goals, the therapist must have goals in mind to prevent the therapy from floundering. The two case examples in Chapter 5 and the case in Chapter 8 provide illustrations of the brief family therapy method as used with confused (sub)systems or families that were unable to focus on specific, concrete goals.

The reframing map (Chapters 3 and 5) can help the therapist to describe what it is that is going on in such a way that developing the different angle seen as necessary for change is possible. Although this mapping technique is the basic "behind-the-mirror technique," it can also be used to describe initiating the reframing-transforming process (represented by the dashed lines) shown on the balance theoretical maps. Although the maps *can* be combined in this way, thinking about this complexity can be more confusing than useful. However, in the actual practice of brief family therapy, the aspects of the situation described with these tools are simultaneous. However, a methodological boundary needs to be drawn somewhere so that the descriptions of a complex process are possible. It is important to remember that these two mapping techniques do not have an "either-or" relationship. Rather, their relationship is more of the "both-and" type. The separation is necessary for clarity of description.

However, that is not an end to the complexity. The decision tree (Chapter 4) can help the therapist focus on the ongoing interactional nature of the suprasystem. The family's response report is a communication about its way of cooperating. That is, in a change or goal-directed therapy, the sequence of "intervention-response report-intervention, and so on," informs the therapist about effectiveness and usefulness. Thus, this descriptive tool is also used simultaneously with the balance theoretical maps that describe the goal and with the reframing maps that describe the family from a different angle. Once again, it is not a matter of this map or that map. Rather, it is *all three maps* that serve *in combination* to guide the therapeutic effort.

Of course, the same methodological reason or descriptive reason meant that the concurrent concepts of isomorphism and cooperating were presented separately. The mapping tools, meant to operationalize the concepts, reflect the "both-and" nature of the concepts. In each message described in the case examples, the two concepts can be seen to apply. The relationship between the two concepts is a "greater-lesser" relationship not an "either-or" relationship.

The intervention designing process can be described as primarily guided by the concept of isomorphism in the case examples in Chapter 5 and Chapter 8. That is, the family's unique manner of cooperating as shown to the team does not indicate that tasks will be useful in promoting change. Therefore, the team will rely more on its descriptions of the family's beliefs about itself (its frames), which it will describe from a different angle when designing the intervention.

Similarly, when the family's manner of cooperating as shown to the team includes task performance (straightforward, modified, or opposite), then the team will rely more on the cooperating concept to guide the development of the interventions (see cases in Chapters 4, 6, and 7). Again, these "task-oriented" change processes and the interventions are not without the guidance of the concept of isomorphism. The task needs to be built upon the team's isomorphic description of the behavioral sequence, and the compliment that precedes the task assignments needs to be isomorphic enough to prompt the development of the "yes set."

In short, the cooperating concept can be seen to guide the task-oriented change process. In these situations the reframing provides news of a difference that makes the new behavior invited by the task possible. The new behavior is more focused because of the task and thus is more directly goal oriented. The isomorphism concept can be seen to guide the "perceptually oriented change process." That is, the reframing provides the news of a difference, and the behavioral proof of this—a change in behavior—is more random.

The descriptive tools, the intervention-designing techniques, the method of delivering a therapeutic message (in two parts: compliment and clue), all reflect the complex nature of the ecosystemic view. The multiple descriptions and explanations on various levels are necessary when dealing with circular systems. Since the ecosystem is circular, the conceptual scheme must also be circular. This emphasis cannot be too strong; none of these descriptions, explanations, or methods should be seen as involved with other descriptions, explanations, or methods in an "either-or" type of relationship.

There can be no escape from the paranoia of the either/or to the "more or less" of the both-and relationships of the rational ecosystem, without the most fundamental changes in values we can conceive of—and perhaps changes even more fundamental than we can actually conceive. (71, p. 228)

All of this complexity reflects the nature of systems, or ecosystems, and the multicausal nature of structural change in these systems. Since a change in one relationship of a system effects the other relationships, and a change in one element of a system effects the other elements, the method of promoting therapeutic change is necessarily complex. When the various levels of the system (cognitive, behavioral, etc.) are also seen as "being in communication," then the necessity for concurrent concepts, such as isomorphism and cooperating, is clear. The two concepts can be seen simultaneously to "aim at" different levels of systemic organization.

Thus, the binocular theory of change, as applied in brief family therapy, can be seen to fit the nature of systems by promoting change on different levels. Systemically, any "effects" can have multiple "causes," and thus the systemic nature of the theory is evident. In fact, the ecosystemic nature of the theory is also evident because the two angles are created by the two subsystems' descriptions of the same data (the family's patterns).

•   •   •

Murphy's Law: "If Anything Can Go Wrong, It Will." Every therapy session, and every sequence of therapy sessions with a particular family, can be seen as experiments with many unknown and unknowable variables. Particularly when the interval between sessions is included in the description, the difficulty of knowing if therapy is effective becomes immense. A therapeutic model needs to be able to make the interconnections between the interventions and change conceptually, otherwise the whole situation is meaningless. A particular model can only guide the therapist along what seems to have been useful trails through this maze of compelxity that are ecosystems. Certainly, the therapy team does not always have success in helping families solve their puzzles or change. Murphy's Law is *always* in effect, no matter how viable the procedures involved.

Since brief family has strong roots in a model of therapy that uses tasks to promote change, the decision tree was developed for the team's use when the "tried and true" tasks did not promote change in a particular situation. In essence, the tree is an attempt to *use* Murphy's Law to the advantage of the family. However, things can *appear* to go wrong (like the first three sessions of the prototype in Chapter 5), which can lead to learning something new and valuable. Therefore, the "experimenter" or therapist needs to worry that: "If Several Things That Could Have Gone Wrong Have Not Gone Wrong, It Would Have Been Ultimately Beneficial For Them To Have Gone Wrong."

References

1. Andolfi, M. *Family therapy: An interactional approach.* New York: Plenum, 1979.
2. Bandler, R., & Grinder, J. *Patterns of the hypnotic techniques of Milton H. Erickson, M.D.* Cupertino, Calif.: Meta, 1975.
3. Bandler, R., & Grinder, J. *The structure of magic.* Palo Alto: Science & Behavior Books, 1975.
4. Bateson, G., & Ruesch, J. *Communication: The social matrix of psychiatry.* New York: Norton, 1951.
5. Bateson, G., Jackson, D. D., Haley, J., & Weakland, J. Toward a theory of schizophrenia. *Behavioral Science* 1:251-264, 1956.
6. Bateson, G., Jackson, D. D., Haley, J., & Weakland, J. A note on the double bind—1962. *Family Process* 2:154-161, 1963.
7. Bateson, G. *Steps to an ecology of mind.* New York: Ballantine, 1972.
8. Bateson, G. The birth of a matrix or double bind and epistemology. In M. Berger (Ed.), *Beyond the double bind.* New York: Brunner/Mazel, 1978.
9. Bateson, G. *Mind and nature.* New York: Dutton, 1979.
10. Beahrs, J. Integrating Erickson's approach. *American Journal of Clinical Hypnosis* 21:55-68, 1977.
11. Boyd, J., Covington, T., Stanaszek, W., & Coussons, J. Drug defaulting. Part 1: Determinants of compliance. *American Journal of Hospital Pharmacology* 31:363-67, 1974.
12. Buckley, W. *Sociology and modern systems theory,* Englewood Cliffs, N.J.: Prentice-Hall, 1967.
13. Capra, F. *The Tao of physics.* New York: Bantam, 1977.
14. Cartwright, D., & Harary, F. Structural balance: A generalization of Heider's theory. *Psychological Review* 63:277-293, 1956.
15. Coyne, J., & Segel, L. A brief, strategic interactional approach to psychotherapy. In J. Anchin & D. Kiesler (Eds.), *Handbook of interpersonal psychotherapy.* New York: Pergamon, 1980.
16. Dell, P. *Beyond homeostasis: Toward a concept of coherence.* Unpublished manuscript, 1980.
17. Dell, P. Some irreverent thoughts on paradox. *Family Process* 20:37-42, 1981.
18. de Shazer, S. The confusion technique. *Family Therapy* 2:23-30, 1975.
19. de Shazer, S. Brief therapy: Two's company. *Family Process* 14:79-93, 1975.
20. de Shazer, S. Brief therapy with couples. *International Journal of Family Counseling* 6:17-30, 1978.
21. de Shazer, S. On transforming symptoms: An approach to an Erickson procedure. *American Journal of Clinical Hypnosis* 22:17-28, 1979.
22. de Shazer, S. Brief therapy with families. *American Journal of Family Therapy* 7:83-95, 1979.
23. de Shazer, S. Investigation of indirect symbolic suggestions. *American Journal of Clinical Hypnosis* 23:10-15, 1980.

24. de Shazer, S. Brief family therapy: A metaphorical task. *Journal of Marital and Family Therapy* **6:**471-476, 1980.
25. Dunlap, K. A revision of the fundamental law of habit formation. *Science* **67:**360-362, 1928.
26. Erickson, M. H. Hypnotic approaches to therapy. *American Journal of Clinical Hypnosis* **20:** 20-35, 1977.
27. Erickson, M. H., & Rossi, E. *Hypnotherapy: An exploratory casebook.* New York: Irvington, 1979.
28. Erickson, M. H., Rossi, E., & Rossi, S. *Hypnotic realities.* New York: Irvington, 1976.
29. Frankl, V. *The doctor and the soul.* New York: Knopf, 1957.
30. Frankl, V. Paradoxical intention. *American Journal of Psychotherapy* **14:**520-535, 1960.
31. Goffman, E. *Frame analysis.* New York: Harper, 1974.
32. Haley, J. An interactional explanation of hypnosis. In D. D. Jackson (Ed.), *Therapy, communication and change.* Palo Alto: Science & Behavior Books, 1968.
33. Haley, J. The family of the schizophrenic: A model system. *Journal of Nervous and Mental Disease* **129:**357-373, 1959.
34. Haley, J. *Strategies of psychotherapy.* New York: Grune & Stratton, 1963.
35. Haley, J. (Ed.). *Advanced techniques of hypnosis and therapy: Selected papers of Milton H. Erickson, M.D.* New York: Grune & Stratton, 1967.
36. Haley, J., & Hoffman, L. *Techniques of family therapy.* New York: Basic Books, 1967.
37. Haley, J. *Uncommon therapy: The psychiatric techniques of Milton H. Erickson, M.D.* New York: Norton, 1973.
38. Haley, J. *Problem-solving therapy.* San Francisco: Jossey-Bass, 1976.
39. Haley, J. Ideas which handicap therapists. In M. Berger (Ed.), *Beyond the double bind.* New York: Brunner/Mazel, 1978.
40. Haley, J. *Leaving home.* New York: McGraw-Hill, 1979.
41. Heider, F. Attitudes and cognitive organization. *Journal of Psychology* **21:**107-112, 1946.
42. Hoffman, L. Deviation-amplifying processes in natural groups. In J. Haley (Ed.), *Changing families.* New York: Grune & Stratton, 1971.
43. Hofstadter, D. *Godel, Escher, Bach: An eternal golden braid.* New York: Basic Books, 1979.
44. Jackson, D. D. The question of family homeostasis. *Psychiatric Quarterly* **31:**79-90, 1957.
45. Jackson, D. D., & Weakland, J. Conjoint family therapy: Some considerations on theory, techniques and results. *Psychiatry* **24:**30-45, 1961.
46. Jackson, D. D. A suggestion for the technical handling of paranoid patients. *Psychiatry* **26:** 306-307, 1963.
47. Keeney, B. Ecosystemic epistemology: An alternative paradigm for diagnosis. *Family Process* **18:**117-129, 1979.
48. Maruyama, M. The second cybernetics: Deviation-amplifying mutual casual processes. *American Scientist* **5:**164-179, 1963.
49. Minuchin, S. *Families and family therapy.* Cambridge: Harvard University Press, 1974.
50. Montalvo, B. Aspects of live supervision. *Family Process* **12:**343-359, 1972.
51. Papp, P. The family that had all the answers. In P. Papp (Ed.), *Family therapy: Full-length case studies.* New York: Gardner, 1977.
52. Rabkin, R. *Strategic psychotherapy.* New York: Basic Books, 1977.
53. Scheflen, A. Communicational concepts of schizophrenia. In M. Berger (Ed.), *Beyond the double bind.* New York: Brunner/Mazel, 1978.
54. Selvini-Palazzoli, M., Boscolo, L., Cecchin, G., & Prata, G. The treatment of children through the brief therapy of the parents. *Family Process* **13:**429-442, 1974.
55. Selvini-Palazzoli, M. *Self-starvation.* New York, Aronson, 1978.
56. Selvini-Palazzoli, M., Boscolo, L., Cecchin, G., & Prata, G. *Paradox and counterparadox.* New York: Aronson, 1973.
57. Selvini-Palazzoli, M., Boscolo, L., Cecchin, G., & Prata, G. A ritualized prescription in family

therapy. *Journal of Marriage and Family Counseling* **4**:3–9, 1978.

58. Soper, P., & L'Abate, L. Paradox as a therapeutic technique. *International Journal of Family Counseling* **5**:10–21, 1977.

59. Speer, D. C. Family systems: Morphostasis and morphogenesis, Or "is homeostasis enough?". *Family Process* **9**:259–278, 1970.

60. Spencer-Brown, G. *Laws of form.* New York: Dutton, 1979.

61. Watts, A. *Psychotherapy East and West.* New York: Vintage, 1961.

62. Watzlawick, P., Beavin, J., & Jackson, D. D. *Pragmatics of human communication.* New York: Norton, 1967.

63. Watzlawick, P. A review of the double bind theory. In D. D. Jackson (Ed.), *Communication, family and marriage.* Palo Alto: Science & Behaviors Books, 1968.

64. Watzlawick, P., Weakland, J., & Fisch, R. *Change.* New York: Norton, 1974.

65. Watzlawick, P., & Coyne, J. Depression following stroke: Brief, problem-focused family treatment. *Family Process* **19**:13–18, 1980.

66. Weakland, J. The "double bind theory" by self-reflexive hindsight. *Family Process* **13**:259–277, 1974.

67. Weakland, J., Fisch, R., Watzlawick, P., & Bodin, A. Brief therapy: Focused problem resolution. *Family Process* **13**:141–168, 1974.

68. Weeks, G., & L'Abate, L. A bibliography of paradoxical methods. *Family Process* **17**:95–98, 1973.

69. Weeks, G., & L'Abate, L. A compilation of paradoxical methods. *American Journal of Family Therapy* **7**:61–76, 1979.

70. Wildon, A. *System and structure.* London: Tavistock, 1972.

71. Wildon, A. *System and structure* (2nd ed.). London: Tavistock, 1980.

Index

Italicized page numbers indicate illustrative examples.